Comprehensive Models of Autism Spectrum Disorder Treatment

Raymond G. Romanczyk • John McEachin
Editors

Comprehensive Models of Autism Spectrum Disorder Treatment

Points of Divergence and Convergence

Springer

Editors
Raymond G. Romanczyk
Institute of Child Development
Binghamton University
Binghamton, NY, USA

John McEachin
Autism Partnership
Seal Beach, CA, USA

ISBN 978-3-319-40903-0 ISBN 978-3-319-40904-7 (eBook)
DOI 10.1007/978-3-319-40904-7

Library of Congress Control Number: 2016948210

Printed on acid-free paper

This Springer imprint is published by Springer Nature
The registered company is Springer International Publishing AG Switzerland

Preface

This book represents the proceedings of a conference held in January 2015 entitled: *Evidence and Rationales for Comprehensive Models of Autism Spectrum Disorder Treatment: Divergence and Convergence*. The conference was a collaboration between the Council on Autism Services and the Autism Partnership, conceived to move forward a critical dialog on the state of autism services. The project spanned 2 years from inception to planning to execution. The conference was very successful and filled to capacity. Thus this was the motivation to bring the proceedings to those who were not fortunate enough to attend.

We have kept the language and tone of the proceedings faithful to the actual presentations. Some adjustment was required because video examples were used in some cases. We also have inserted references into the text although these were not all part of the actual presentations. We did this to allow the reader further resources as a substitute for the conversations that took place at the conference when attendees wished further information.

Of note, the presenters all shared their knowledge gratis—there were no speaker stipends or honoraria. They spoke because of their commitment to the filed of autism spectrum disorder which in turn allowed us to produce a conference that did not present a financial barrier to those many individuals who wanted to attend. The detailed, innovative, evidence-based, and collegial presentations and discussions presented here represent a unique and much needed addition to the professional and consumer literature.

I wish to thank all of my colleagues at the Council on Autism Services (recently had a name change to Council of Autism Service Providers—CASP) and the Autism Partnership for supporting this effort, our speakers who gave so graciously of their time, knowledge, and expertise, and I also want to thank Dr. Rachel Cavalari who worked tirelessly with me to make the conference and the proceedings come to fruition.

Binghamton, NY — Raymond G. Romanczyk

Preface

Acknowledgments

We thank Jennifer Bertolo for her excellent assistance in the initial transcript editing and the integration of the presenters' graphics with the conference transcripts.

Contents

Contents

Contributors

William H. Ahearn, Ph.D., BCBA-D The New England Center for Children, Southborough, MA, USA

Rachel N.S. Cavalari, Ph.D., BCBA-D Institute for Child Development, Binghamton University, Binghamton, NY, USA

Jennifer M. Gillis, Ph.D., BCBA-D Binghamton University, Binghamton, NY, USA

Ronald Leaf, Ph.D. Autism Partnership, Seal Beach, CA, USA

Sally Rogers, Ph.D. UC Davis, Mind Institute, Davis, CA, USA

Mark L. Sundberg, Ph.D., BCBA-D Behavior Analysis Center for Autism, Fishers, IN, USA

About the Contributors

William H. Ahearn, Ph.D., BCBA-D, joined The New England Center for Children in August 1996 and currently serves at NECC as the Director of Research. He is also Adjunct Faculty in Western New England University's doctoral and masters programs. He was the 2009 American Psychological Association—Division 25 awardee for Enduring Contributions to Applied Behavioral Research. He has published extensively on behavior analytic interventions for treating problem behavior and teaching social and communicative behavior for individuals with autism, related disabilities, and typically developing children. Dr. Ahearn is Past President of the Association of Professional Behavior Analysts and the Berkshire Association for Behavior Analysis and Therapy, has been involved in establishing regulatory practices for behavior analysts, and currently serves on the Massachusetts Board that licenses behavior analysts. He also serves as Editor-in-Chief for Behavioral Interventions and sits on the Editorial Boards of several other journals.

Rachel N.S. Cavalari, Ph.D., BCBA-D, is a New York Licensed Psychologist and Licensed Behavior Analyst, at the Institute for Child Development at Binghamton University. She is an Adjunct Professor in the Department of Psychology and also serves as Practicum Liaison and Coordinating Instructor for the Undergraduate Psychology Major Track in Applied Behavior Analysis and as the BACB Approved Continuing Education Coordinator. Her current interests include staff training, behavioral assessment and intervention, diagnostic evaluation, systems analysis, and regulation and practice issues for clinicians. Dr. Cavalari received her doctorate in Clinical Psychology from Binghamton University in 2012. Dr. Cavalari served on the Board of Directors for the New York State Association for Behavior Analysis from 2013 to 2014 and has since served on the NYSABA Legislative Committee.

Jennifer M. Gillis, Ph.D., BCBA-D, is an Associate Professor of Psychology and the Associate Director of the Institute for Child Development at Binghamton University. She serves as Co-Director of the Undergraduate Psychology Major Track in Applied Behavior Analysis. Dr. Gillis is an Adjunct Assistant Professor at

Upstate Medical University. Her professional and research interests include the training of clinicians, behavior analysts, and caregivers, assessment and treatment of autism spectrum disorders, and development and evaluation of systems of data collection and analysis. Dr. Gillis received her doctorate in Clinical Psychology from Binghamton University, after completing her predoctoral internship at Alpert Medical School of Brown University. From 2006 to 2012 she was an Associate Professor in the Psychology Department at Auburn University. Dr. Gillis previously served as the Executive Director for the Alabama Association for Behavior Analysis and continues to remain active in issues related to policy and dissemination.

Ronald Leaf, Ph.D. , is a licensed psychologist who has over 40 years of experience in the field of Autism Spectrum Disorder. He began his career working with Ivar Lovaas while receiving his undergraduate degree at UCLA, subsequently receiving his doctorate under the direction of Dr. Lovaas. During his years at UCLA he served as Clinic Supervisor, Research Psychologist, Interim Director of the Autism Project, and Lecturer. He was extensively involved in several research investigations, contributed to the Me Book, and is a coauthor of the Me Book Videotapes, a series of instructional tapes for teaching autistic children. Dr. Leaf has consulted to families, schools, day programs, and residential facilities on a national and international basis and presently serves as Director of Autism Partnership. Dr. Leaf has published extensively in research journals and is the coauthor of *A Work in Progress*, *Time for School*, *It Has to Be Said!*, *Crafting Connections*, and *A Work in Progress Companion Series*.

Sally Rogers, Ph.D. , is a developmental psychologist, clinician, Professor of Psychiatry and Behavioral Sciences, and Director of Training and Mentoring at the MIND Institute, University of California Davis. She has been the principal investigator of several NIH-funded multi-site autism research projects, including a 10-year CPEA program project and two funded Autism Centers of Excellence (ACE) network projects. She has served as president of the International Society for Autism Research, associate editor of the journal *Autism Research*, a member of the Autism Speaks Global Autism Public Health Initiative, a fellow of the American Psychological Association, Division 33, and a member of the Autism, PDD, and other Developmental Disorders workgroup for the DSM 5. The Early Start Denver Model that she developed with Geri Dawson and other colleagues at the University of Colorado Health Sciences Center, the University of Washington, and the University of California Davis is internationally known and recognized by Time.com and Autism Speaks as one of the ten most important scientific findings of 2012.

Mark Sundberg, Ph.D., BCBA-D , is a licensed psychologist with over 40 years of clinical experience who consults for public and private schools that serve children with autism. He received his doctorate degree in Applied Behavior Analysis from Western Michigan University (1980), under the direction of Dr. Jack Michael. He is the author of the Verbal Behavior Milestones Assessment and Placement Program (VB-MAPP) and coauthored the ABLLS and the book *Teaching Language* *to Children with Autism or Other Developmental Disabilities*. He is the founder and past editor of the journal *The Analysis of Verbal Behavior*, twice past president of The Northern California Association for Behavior Analysis, past chair of the Publication Board of ABAI, and has served on the Board of Directors of the B. F. Skinner Foundation. Dr. Sundberg has given hundreds of national and international conference presentations and taught 80 college and university courses on behavior analysis, verbal behavior, sign language, and child development. In 2013, he received the "Jack Michael Outstanding Contributions in Verbal Behavior Award" from ABAI's Verbal Behavior Special Interest Group.

About the Editors

John McEachin is a behavior analyst and licensed psychologist who has been providing intervention to children with autism as well as adolescents and adults with a wide range of developmental disabilities since 1977. He received his graduate training under Professor Ivar Lovaas at UCLA on the Young Autism Project. During his 11 years at UCLA, Dr. McEachin served in various roles including Clinic Supervisor, Research Assistant, and Teaching Assistant. His research has included the long-term follow-up study of the participants in the Young Autism Project, which was published in 1993. In 1994 he joined with Ron Leaf in forming Autism Partnership, which they co-direct. In 1999 they published *A Work in Progress*, a widely used behavioral treatment manual and curriculum for children with autism. Dr. McEachin has lectured throughout the world and coauthored numerous books and research articles. He consults regularly to families, agencies, and school districts, assisting in the development of treatment programs and providing training to parents, group home staff, and classroom personnel.

Raymond G. Romanczyk is a SUNY Distinguished Service Professor in the Clinical Psychology program at Binghamton University. He is a NY Licensed Behavior Analyst, NY Licensed Clinical Psychologist, and a Board Certified Behavior Analyst—Doctoral and received his Ph.D. from Rutgers University. In addition, Dr. Romanczyk is an Adjunct Professor of Psychiatry of the SUNY Health Sciences Center of Syracuse. Dr. Romanczyk is the founder and director of the Institute for Child Development that has been providing clinical and educational services to children and families for 40 years, and is one of ten programs cited in the Educating Children with Autism report of the National Research Council.

He is a Fellow of the American Psychological Association and he is a founding board member of the Association of Professional Behavior Analysts, was a member of the scientific advisory board of the National Autism Center, and a founding board member of the Council on Autism Services, a national organization of directors of autism service agencies. He is a consultant to the NYS Department of Health Early Intervention Program and was a panel member on the NYSDOH clinical guidelines for autism, one of the first empirically based reviews of autism assessment and treatment practices. He also serves as an associate editor and member of the editorial board and reviewer for numerous professional journals. Recent published works include “Efficacy of Behavioral Interventions for Young Children with Autism Spectrum Disorders: Public Policy, the Evidence Base, and Implementation Parameters” and “The Status of Treatment for Autism Spectrum Disorders: The Weak Relationship of Science to Interventions.” Dr. Romanczyk has presented several hundred addresses at regional, national, and international professional conferences regarding his applied and research work at the Institute and has received numerous awards for his clinical and research accomplishments.

Chapter 1
Prologue and Introduction

Raymond G. Romanczyk

Autism spectrum disorder is a complex, multiply expressed disorder of the core of human functioning—social interaction. Leo Kanner (Kanner, 1943) first identified the syndrome of autism in the early 1940s, using the term "early infantile autism" to connote his assertion that this was a disorder that was present from birth. Importantly, of the many characteristics Kanner described, the most important was the characterization of aloof, highlighting the core deficit in social interaction. While Kanner's initial publication described only 11 children, he set the stage for further examination of this, at the time, rare disorder. For decades the prevalence for autism was in the 4.5 per 10,000 range as would be expected for a rare disorder. There were of course some differences in various estimates of prevalence, from a low of 2 per 10,000 to a high of 13.9 per 10,000, but all in this very low prevalence range. Then in the late 1990s, estimates began to rise.

The California Department of Developmental Services reported in 1999 a prevalence of 20 per 10,000. Some of the reporting at the time distorted the magnitude of change by reporting the figure as 1 per 500 that had more impact on perception of increase than the standard per 10,000 method. This could be viewed as the start of the autism "epidemic." In rapid succession, reported prevalence began a steady climb. This pattern is in parallel to standards for diagnosis and follows a clear pattern (Romanczyk, Turner, Sevlever, & Gillis, 2014). Autism was first introduced into formal psychiatric diagnosis in the Diagnostic and Statistical Manual (DSM),

R.G. Romanczyk (✉)
Institute for Child Development, Binghamton University, Vestal Parkway East, Binghamton, NY 13902, USA
e-mail: rromanc@binghamton.edu

R.G. Romanczyk, J. McEachin (eds.), *Comprehensive Models of Autism Spectrum Disorder Treatment*, DOI 10.1007/978-3-319-40904-7_1

version III, of the American Psychiatric Association in 1980 under Kanner's term "infantile autism." Six characteristics were required:

1. Onset before 30 months of age
2. A pervasive lack of responsiveness to other people
3. Gross deficits in language development
4. When speech is present, peculiar speech patterns such as immediate and delayed echolalia, metaphorical language, and pronoun reversal
5. Bizarre responses to various aspects of the environment (e.g., resistance to change, peculiar interest in or attachments to objects)
6. The absence of delusions, hallucinations, loosening of associations, and incoherence as observed in individuals diagnosed with schizophrenia

Relatively quickly, in 1987, DSM-III was revised, DSM-III-R, with significant changes. The characteristics required were reduced to three:

1. Impairment in reciprocal social interaction
2. Impairment in verbal and nonverbal communication
3. Restrictive repertoire of activities and interests

Within these three categories were numerous specific examples of symptoms, with at least half required, in a specific pattern, to make the diagnosis. In like manner, in 1994 DSM-IV was released with modifications to the criteria and so again in 2000 with DSM-IV-TR. The basic structure of the three core categories remained, but with changes in specific requirements. The last revision, DSMV in 2013, was a profound change from previous versions. No longer were there separate diagnostic categories of autistic disorder, Asperger's disorder, and pervasive developmental disability—not otherwise specified. Rather, there was one diagnostic category of autism spectrum disorder. Further, the number of symptom categories was reduced from three to two:

1. Persistent deficit in social communication and social interaction
2. Restricted, repetitive patterns of behavior, interests, or activities

However, it is now the case that all three symptom examples listed for category one must be met, and two of the symptom examples in category two must be met, significantly reducing the number of permutations of symptom combinations. Some researchers have commented on whether the DSM-V change will be positive or negative for services (e.g., Dawson, 2012; Lord et al., 2011; McPartland, Reichow, & Volkmar, 2012), but the full impact of these changes in DSM-V will not be understood fully for a number of years.

Given this perspective, it is important to note that the CDC currently estimates a prevalence of 1 in 68—http://www.cdc.gov/media/releases/2014/p0327-autism-spectrum-disorder.html. This is an extraordinary change from the historic 4.5 per 10,000. While there are certainly important questions to be answered about the increase in prevalence, such as change in diagnostic criteria, it is not central to our purpose. Thus, whatever the reason for the current very high prevalence, and because of the specific characteristics of ASD, with its wide variation in expression of symptoms and variation in impairment to language, cognition, and adaptive behavior, ASD stands out for the extensive impact it has on the individual, family, caregivers and service providers, the community, and broader society. The costs of providing services are enormous, and many services that are offered are ineffective, adding to the cost burden (Romanczyk, Callahan, Turner, & Cavalari, 2014). No matter what the factors are that are increasing prevalence, the need for services for individuals and families is clear and represents an imperative to provide generally available and evidence-based services to insure all individuals may participate as they and their families wish in effective services.

Somewhat in parallel to the changing diagnostic criteria and prevalence trend has been the change in the right to access services. It is possible to identify school programs for children who would now be diagnosed with ASD back in the mid-1800s. Since that time many such schools have provided services, but until comparatively recently, they were private, not public schools. Well into the later 1900s, children with ASD were routinely deprived of publically funded education. The passing of Public Law 94-142 (Education of All Handicapped Children Act) by Congress in 1975 helped change that widespread practice but only very slowly. By the early 2000s, many more public school programs were available, but very very few could be characterized as providing state-of-the art evidence-based services—that designation remained solidly in the realm of private schools and programs. The same pattern could be said of health insurance coverage for ASD—often lacking and typically inadequate for effective intervention.

The current status has changed quite dramatically, especially with respect to insurance coverage, although funding tension remains in distinguishing medical necessity from a health insurance point of view and education access from a public education right perspective (Romanczyk, Callahan, et al., 2014). There are significant differences state to state across the United States, resulting in both regional and national challenges. However, as access to services and education continues to improve, the focus must be kept on effectiveness of services, not simply access to "something."

Access to effective services can be hampered by a lack of objective information, inadequate funding, lack of trained professionals, and use of popular but ineffective interventions. There are well over 300 interventions for autism, the vast majority of which are not evidence based as effective (Myers & Johnson, 2007; National Autism Center, 2009; National Research Council, 2001; Romanczyk, Gillis, White, & DiGennaro 2008). Within this context of evidence-based versus simply claimed effectiveness, it is clear that there is a substantial body of research supporting behavioral intervention which includes applied behavior analysis (Romanczyk, Callahan, et al., 2014). Even within this small percentage of all interventions that can actually demonstrate effectiveness through controlled research, there are differences in the specifics of implementation. This can cause confusion for consumers as well as legislators, administrators, educators, and other service providers as to the specifics of each approach, its evidence, the specific implementation parameters, and its cost. Too often practitioners and researchers interact primarily with those sharing a similar perspective and in forums that do not allow for clear delineation of similarities and differences. Also, different treatment approaches are often oversimplified in characterizations and at times completely misrepresented. Even the term evidenced based has been corrupted to include opinion and anecdote rather than methodologically sound and rigorous research. It is in this context of great need, great exaggeration, distortion, and limited access to coordinated and detailed presentation and discussion by researcher-clinicians that this proactive conference was convened.

Conference on Evidence and Rationales for Comprehensive Models of Autism Spectrum Disorder Treatment: Points of Divergence and Convergence

All right, so now some perspective. It's clear that efforts to improve the functioning of individuals who have significant skill deficits and significant problems in social interactions have been one of the most fruitful undertakings of the behavioral sciences in the last couple decades—the past five decades. There is overwhelming demand for intervention services—no surprise to any of you all here today. But consumers and practitioners are drawn to various models of services and interventions for a number of reasons. Some are rational; some are emotional. It's not that one is good or bad; it's just that they are very different. And today, what we're going to focus on is some of the conceptual structures and evidence base for models that are effective in producing solid behavior change.

So we're going to do this in a form that is a little different. We were talking about this last night. This is not going to be a "celebrity deathmatch" confrontational event that you sometimes see. No, this is a group who are scientists, practitioners, and colleagues, getting together to discuss, in some depth, their approach, their model, why, how, etc. At the end, we're going to deal with some common issues and problems that we all face. So that's the general setup. We've given the speakers a really difficult task and that is to take everything they've put their heart and soul into for the past few decades and condense it down into an hour. So for this effort we thank them very much.

Now, why is there a need for focus on evidence-based services? Well, one is ASD prevalence. Right? Some of us are old enough to remember when the prevalence was 4.5 in 10,000. As of today, it's estimated as 1 in 68. That's a big change. That's a really big change. Why is there an increase? We could have a conference just on that and that could get very contentious. The theories on that are very striking. And so it begs the questions from consumers: how can we provide treatment services if we don't know the cause? That is an interesting problem, conceptually.

We also have problems, nationally, in equity and availability. Not everyone has equal access to quality services. We also have an interesting debate in this country about what is an educational requirement and what is medically necessary (Romanczyk, Callahan, et al., 2014). Those of you involved in helping families receive services from school districts, insurance, etc., you know these battles. While there is expansion of coverage, and thus more and more individuals are receiving services, at the same time, if we look at it nationally, the services given individual children are constrained. It's the size of the pie problem of resources—as more come in, that means we may see reduction in quality—well, not may. Wait, that was too kind. We are seeing below threshold levels of effective services and I think many consumers don't realize that. And the difficulty with services being sort of a la carte is that there is diversion of limited resources away from evidence-based services to those that don't have an evidence base. This is a societal judgment on how funding should be dispersed. And of course, ineffective services impact the individual, the family, and the society. Again, we could spend a day on each of these topics and barely scratch the surface. The reason we're going over it is just to say that everything you're going to hear today is in a context—a much broader context—but we need a starting point and the starting point for us is, if you will, the evidence base.

And last, it is not simply that access is not sufficient; effectiveness is the requirement. It's not helpful to have access to services that are not going to produce meaningful and substantial change in the long term.

So, what is our structure? Each speaker will have 1 h to address the following issues:

1. An overview of the approach
2. The conceptual basis for the approach
3. The primary procedural components
4. How goals are selected and sequenced
5. Staff skill/training required
6. The evidence base

And we've asked each speaker to address each of these issues to give you all some consistency across presentations and a basis for some comparison. So an overview of the approach, conceptual basis, primary procedural components, how goals are selected and sequenced, staff training that's required, and the evidence base.

And just to let you know, we're really grateful for the speakers because, usually in a conference, you say, "Hey Mark, come on down and do what you want!" So these individuals are used to not getting instructions on exactly what to present. They've been extremely gracious, all of them, in helping us follow this format to allow for a good discussion.

Our focus is on young children because we had to have some focus to constrain this to a one-day conference. Need is also great for discussion about school age, adolescents, young adults, and older adults. It's not that we're ignoring this. We're not. We're just putting it in the perspective of time for a one-day conference. Those will be topics for another time.

Now to our speakers: they really do need no introduction. But if you do want some introduction we have short bios about each of the folks. Because our goal is to give each of them the most amount of time to speak, rather than going through the more standard introduction formalities, we will simply begin. So, let's get started! Ron, I think that's our transition to you.

References

Dawson, G. (2012, June 11). DSM-5 update: Our letter to the revision committee. *Autism Speaks*. Retrievedfromhttp://www.autismspeaks.org/blog/2012/06/11/dsm-5-update-our-letter-revision-committee?&utm_source=social-media&utm_medium=text-link&utm_campaign=espeaks

Kanner, L. (1943). Autistic disturbances of affective contact. *Nervous Child, 2*, 217–250.

Lord, C., Petkova, E., Hus, V., Gan, W., Lu, F., Martin, D., … Risi, S. (2011). A multisite study of the clinical diagnosis of different autism spectrum disorders. *Archives of General Psychiatry, 69*(3), 306–313.

McPartland, J. D., Reichow, B., & Volkmar, F. R. (2012). Sensitivity and specificity of proposed DSM-5 diagnostic criteria for autism spectrum disorder. *Journal of the American Academy of Child and Adolescent Psychiatry, 51*(4), 368–383.

Myers, S., & Johnson, C. P. (2007). Management of children with autism spectrum disorders. *Pediatrics, 120*(5), 1162–1182.

National Autism Center. (2009). *National standards report: National standards project—addressing the need for evidence-based practice guidelines for autism spectrum disorders*. Randolph: National Autism Center.

National Research Council. (2001). In C. Lord & J. P. McGee (Eds.), *Educating children with autism*. Washington: National Academy Press.

Romanczyk, R. G., Callahan, E. H., Turner, L. B., & Cavalari, R. N. S. (2014). Efficacy of behavioral interventions for young children with autism spectrum disorders: Public policy, the evidence base, and implementation parameters. *Review Journal of Autism and Developmental Disorders, 1*, 276–326.

Romanczyk, R. G., Gillis, J. M., White, S., & DiGennaro, F. (2008). Comprehensive treatment packages for ASD: Perceived vs. proven effectiveness. In J. L. Matson (Ed.), *Clinical assessment and intervention for autism spectrum disorders* (pp. 351–381). Burlington, MA: Elsevier.

Romanczyk, R. G., Turner, L. B., Sevlever, M., & Gillis, J. (2014). The status of treatment for autism spectrum disorders: The weak relationship of science to interventions. In S. O. Lilienfeld, J. M. Lohr, & S. J. Lynn (Eds.), *Science and pseudoscience in contemporary clinical psychology*. New York: Guilford.

Chapter 2
"The Lovaas Model: Love It or Hate It, But First Understand It"

Ronald Leaf and John McEachin

I have obsessed over this presentation. My wife and my boys would say I have been possessed. It has given me a chance to reflect, regret, and rejoice my 11-year journey working with Ivar. If it was not for Ivar, I would not be here today. I would not be in the field either. Most likely, I would be chasing ambulances or perhaps become a politician.

I am grateful for the opportunity to be able to clarify and describe my 11-year journey working with Ivar. Because whether you love, hate, or are indifferent to the Lovaas model, it is likely that you may not know exactly what occurred during the Lovaas project.

Unfortunately, there is a tremendous amount of misinformation and misinterpretation of what occurred at UCLA (Leaf & McEachin, 2008). It is one of the reasons why we wrote, *It Has To Be Said* (Leaf, McEachin, & Taubman, 2008). This was the cover that we, well at least I, wanted to use—Lemmings jumping into the sea—but our publisher thought it was slightly offensive (Fig. 2.1).

So we compromised on this cover (Fig. 2.2).

One of the chapters we wrote was devoted to clarifying the Lovaas model (Leaf & McEachin, 2008). The senior members of Autism Partnership felt we needed to fully clarify and describe what occurred during our generation. This is us more recently (Fig. 2.3):

And this was us long ago (Fig. 2.4):

We have been together for a long time, longer than our marriages.

R. Leaf, Ph.D. (✉)
Autism Partnership, 200 Marina Dr., Seal Beach, CA, USA
e-mail: Rlautpar@aol.com

J. McEachin
Autism Partnership, 200 Marina Drive, Seal Beach, CA 90740, USA
e-mail: JMAutPar@aol.com

R.G. Romanczyk, J. McEachin (eds.), *Comprehensive Models of Autism Spectrum Disorder Treatment*, DOI 10.1007/978-3-319-40904-7_2

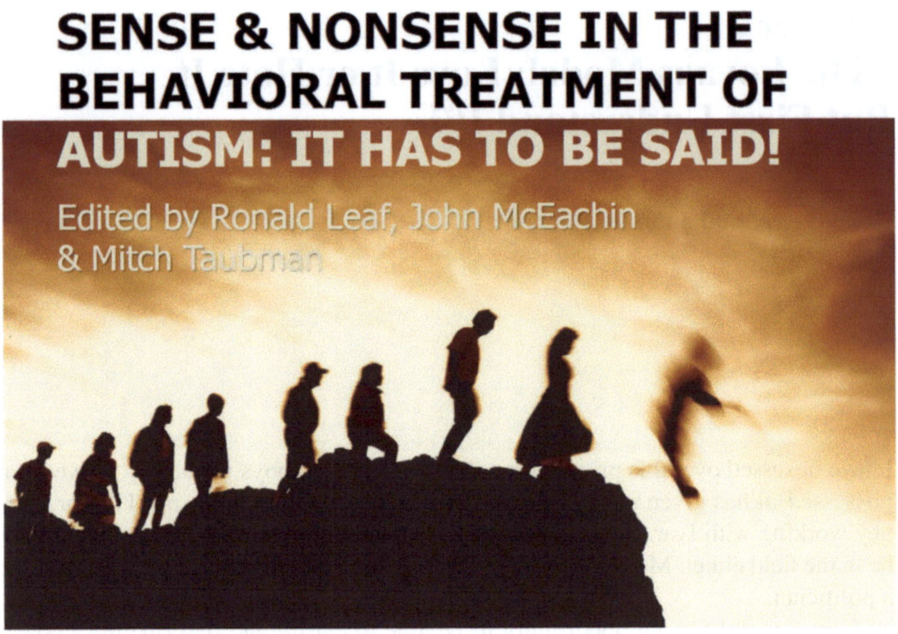

Fig. 2.1 Early draft of book cover, "Sense & Nonsense in the Behavioral Treatment of Autism: It Has to be Said"

Personal History

My journey in Autism started in 1973. I was an undergraduate student, a political science major in my junior year at UCLA. I needed a class on Tuesdays and Thursdays from 2:00 to 3:15. You may ask why that specific day and time? Well because it would allow me to only have to go to school 2 days a week. When I got the schedule of classes I narrowed my choices down to two classes, an art history and a psychology class. I asked my friends the very important question, "What's the easiest class?" They said they were both easy "A's." So now what was I to do? I looked at the location of the classes. UCLA is a big campus so I did not want to walk too far. They were both equally close to my other classes. So before I flipped a coin, I asked my sister-in-law, who was a double major in art history and psychology, for her advice. She asked what the classes were. I said one is Integrated Arts. She approved, saying it was a brilliant class, her favorite class ever at UCLA, and that Professor Kaiser was amazing. She wanted to know what the other class was (Fig. 2.5).

I answered it was Foundations of Behavior Modification; Ivar Lovaas is the professor. She said, "He does evil work. Don't take the class." I was intrigued; I took the class. After the first week, I decided to change my career path. I was captivated by autism and intrigued and inspired by Ivar. That is how I got into the field.

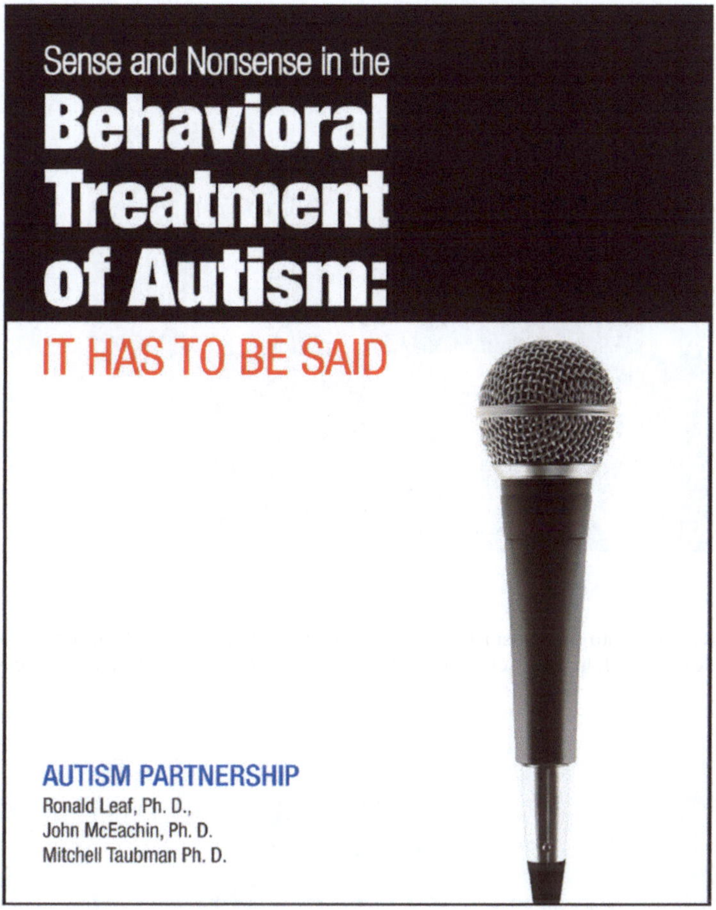

Fig. 2.2 Final version of book cover

An Overview of the Lovaas Model

Nowadays, we hear about the Lovaas model, but I never quite know what that means. Is it the model of the early 1960s, the pioneering days of autism when little was known about autism? (Fig. 2.6)

When children were referred to as being afflicted with childhood psychosis or childhood schizophrenia? When children lived their lives in state institutions? When self-injurious behavior was referred to as self-destructive behavior? Are those the days they were talking about? When Ivar and his army of undergraduate and graduate students did everything they could do to conquer the devastating disorder of autism?

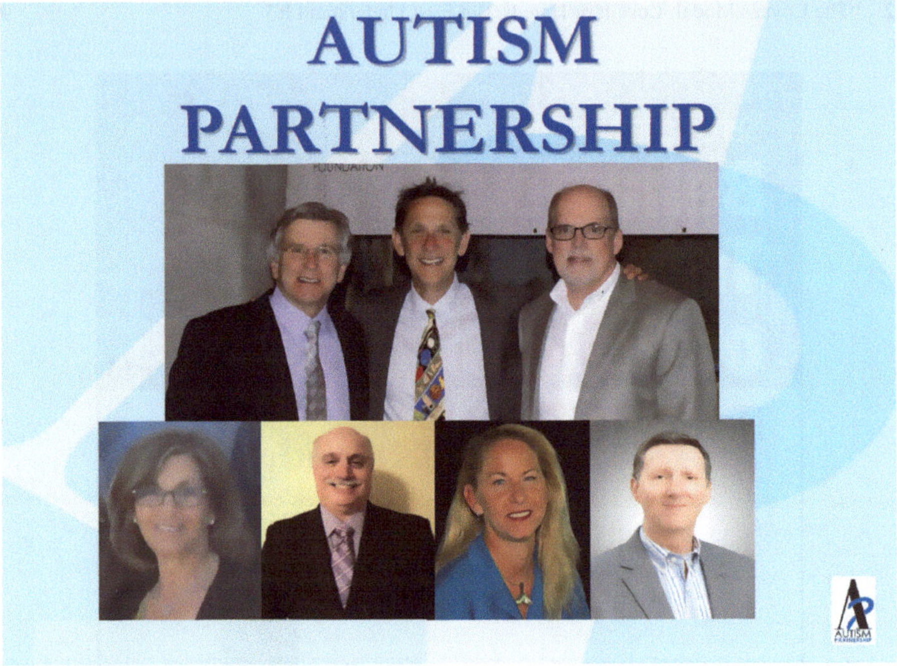

Fig. 2.3 Recent Photo of Autism Partnership Senior Staff (clockwise from upper left): Mitch Taubman, Ron Leaf, John McEachin, Andi Waks, Sandi Slater, Tracee Parker & Marc Mullins

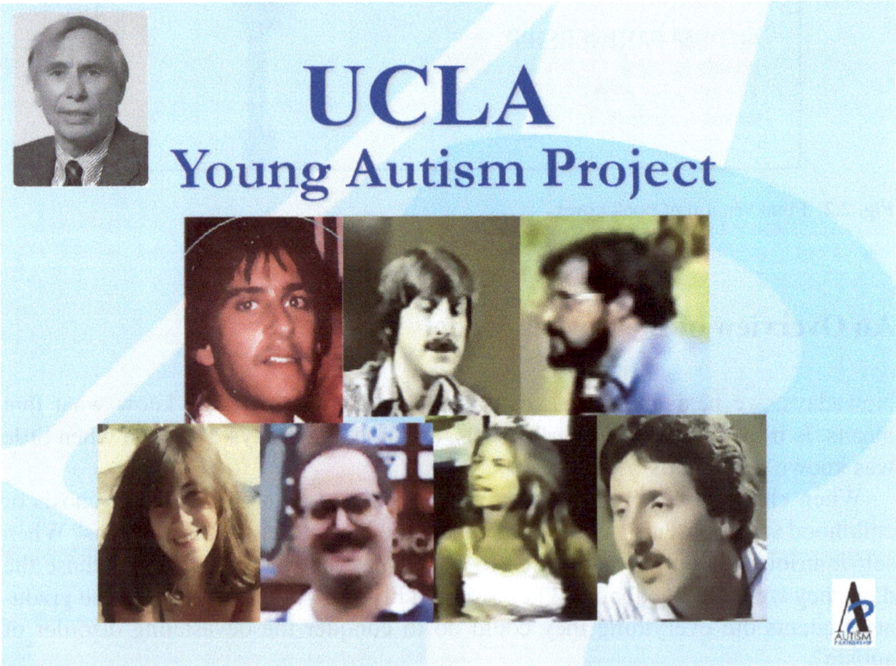

Fig. 2.4 Photo from 1970's

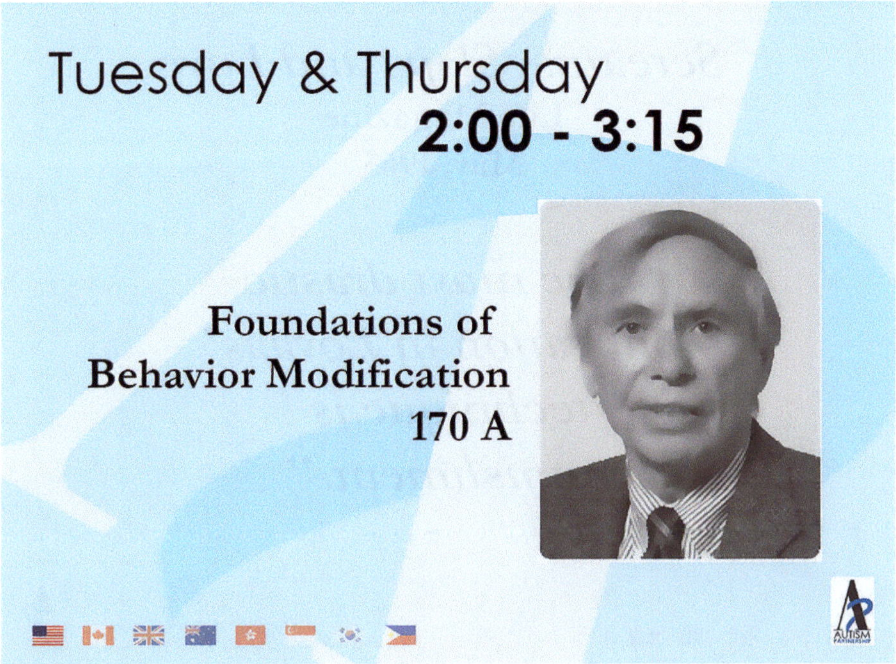
Tuesday & Thursday
2:00 - 3:15
Foundations of
Behavior Modification
170 A
AUTISM

Fig. 2.5 UCLA Course listing for Psychology 170A

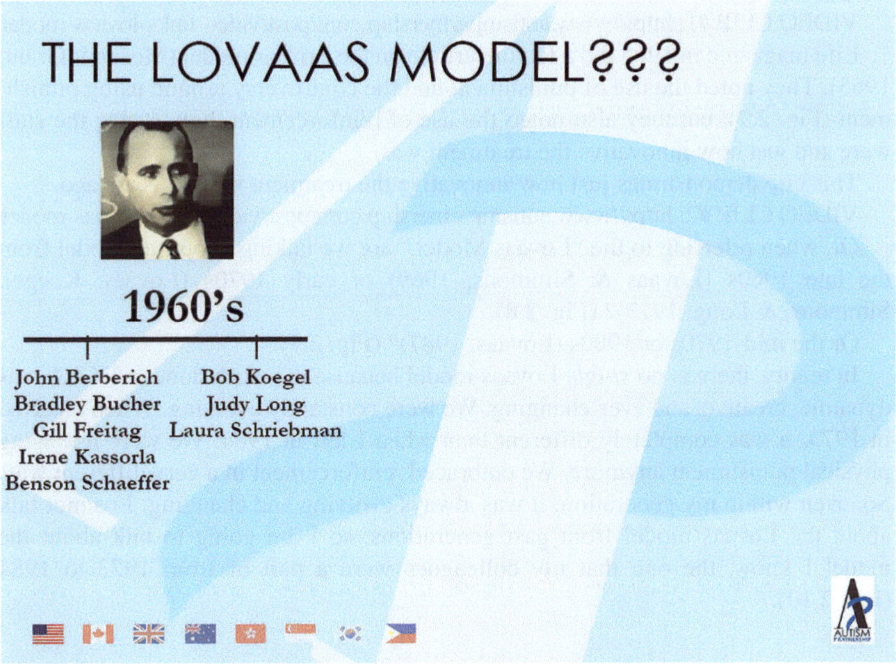

Fig. 2.6 Lovaas Associates during 1960's

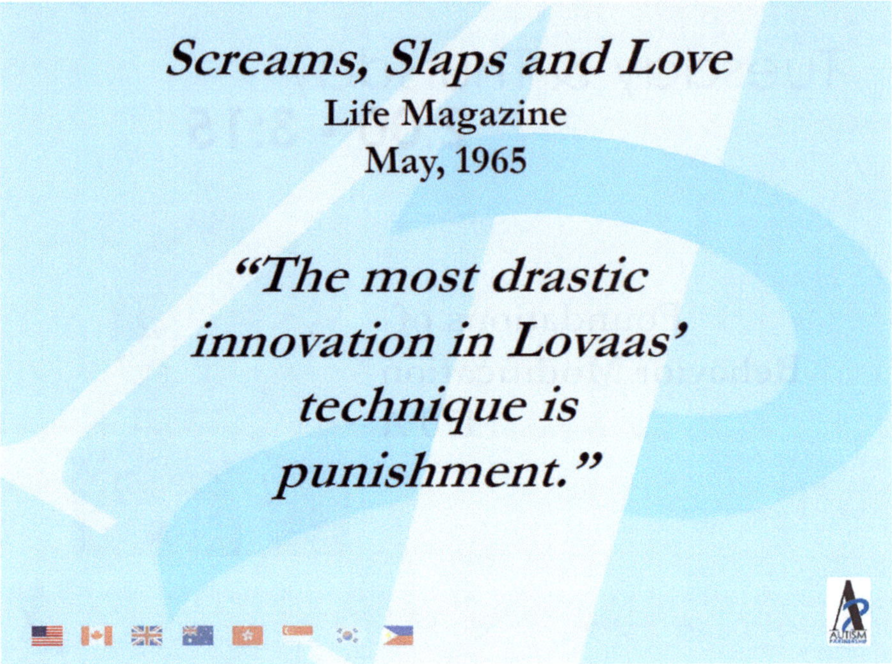

Fig. 2.7 From Life Magazine 1965

VIDEO CLIP #1: http://www.autismpartnership.com/post/video-links-lovaas-model

Life magazine in 1965 did a feature article on the Lovaas model (Moser & Grant, 1965). They noted the use of punishment and the controversy around using punishment (Fig. 2.7), but they also noted the use of reinforcement, how caring the staff were and just how innovative the treatment was.

This clip demonstrates just how innovative the treatment was 50 years ago.

VIDEO CLIP #2: http://www.autismpartnership.com/post/video-links-lovaas-model

Or, when referring to the "Lovaas Model," are we talking about the model from the late 1960s (Lovaas & Simmons, 1969) or early 1970s (Lovaas, Koegel, Simmons, & Long, 1973)? (Fig. 2.8)

Or the mid-1970s or 1980s (Lovaas, 1987)? (Fig. 2.9)

In reality, there is no *single* Lovaas model because the work done at UCLA was dynamic, creative, and ever-changing. We were constantly evolving. When I started in 1973, it was completely different than when I left in 1984. We were not using physical punishment anymore. We embraced reinforcement in a very different way. So, even within my generation, it was always evolving and changing. I cannot talk about the Lovaas model from past generations, so I am going to talk about the model I know, the one that my colleagues were a part of from 1973 to 1984 (Fig. 2.10).

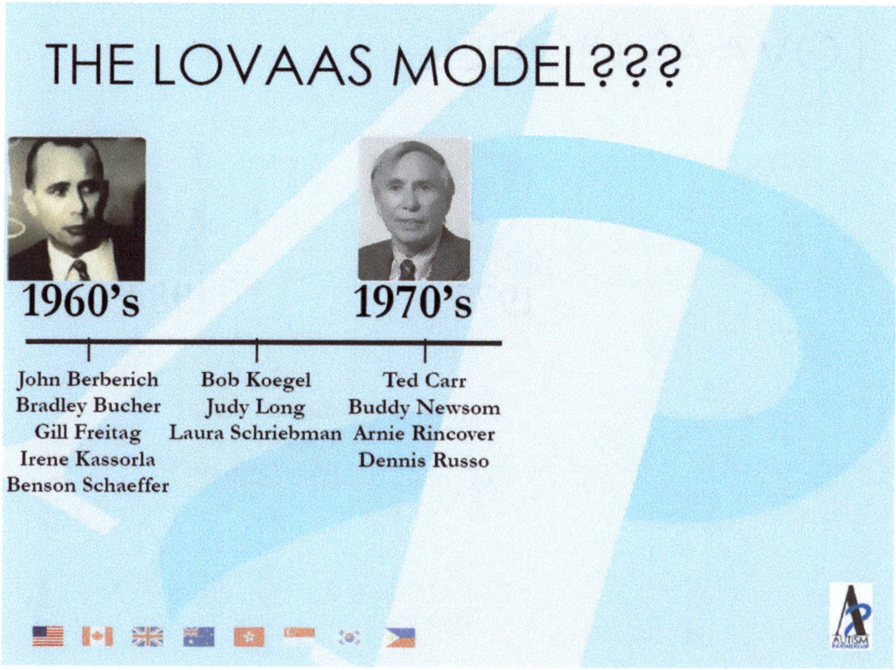

Fig. 2.8 Lovaas Associates during 1970's

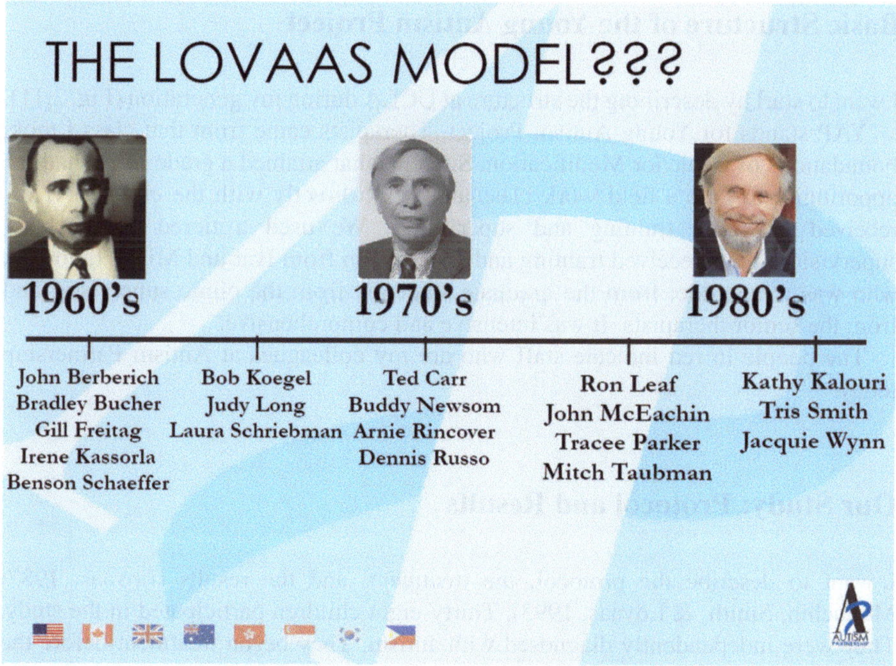

Fig. 2.9 Lovaas Associates during 1980's

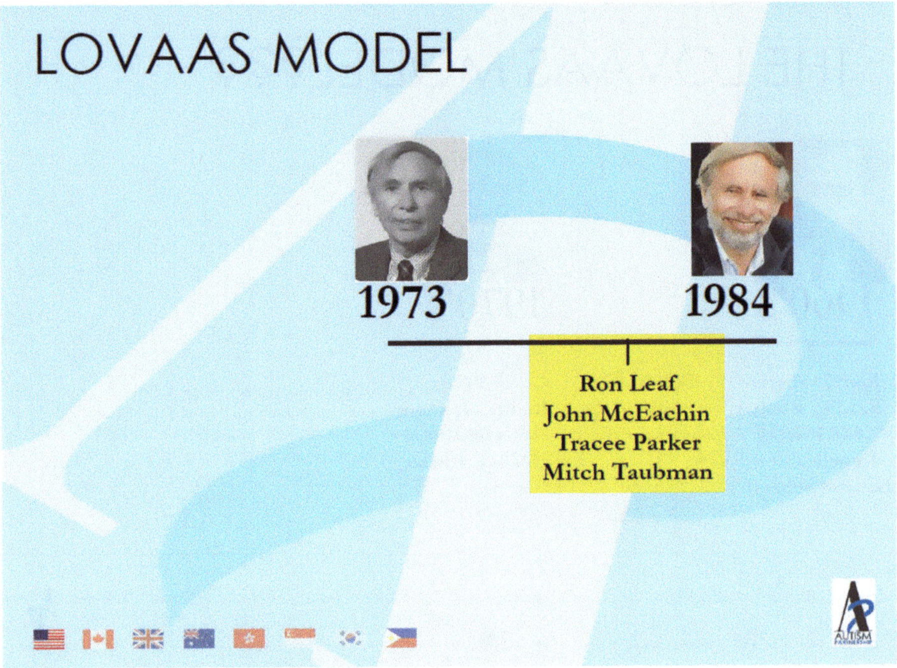

Fig. 2.10 Lovaas Associates during the Leaf and McEachin era

Basic Structure of the Young Autism Project

I want to start by describing the structure at UCLA during my generation (Fig. 2.11).

YAP stands for Young Autism Project. Therapists came from that class I took, Foundations of Behavior Modification. Students that attained a grade of 'A' had the opportunity to take a field work class and work directly with the children. They received extensive training and supervision. We used a tiered approach of supervision. Staff received training and supervision from Ivar and Mitch Taubman, who was a post-doc; from the graduate students; from the clinic supervisor; and from the senior therapists. It was intensive and comprehensive.

The people in red indicate staff who are my colleagues at Autism Partnership today.

Our Study: Protocol and Results

I want to describe the protocol, the treatment, and the results (Lovaas, 1987; McEachin, Smith, & Lovaas, 1993). Thirty-eight children participated in the study. They were independently diagnosed with autism. They began treatment before the

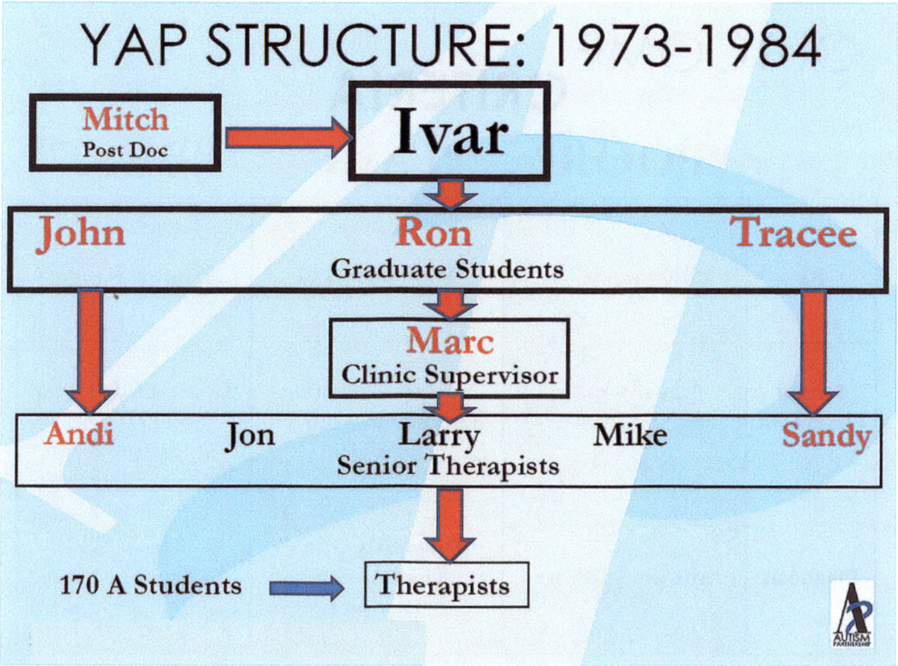

Fig. 2.11 UCLA Young Autism Project Organizational Chart

age of four. Half of the children, 19 of them, received an average of 40 h of ABA weekly. The treatment was broad in scope, encompassing all areas of functioning including language, social, behavior, play, and self-help. We used the principles of ABA to increase desired behaviors and to decrease maladaptive behaviors. Our aim was to have the children engaged in learning and connected with the world around them every minute of the day. The therapy team provided many hours per day of formal intervention. But the rest of the day was equally important and the parents were essential partners in the treatment process. The model was very ambitious, very directive, because the goal was to close the developmental gap. We hypothesized that would only happen if we could speed up the learning process and actively steer the children away from spending their time engaged in narrow interests and repetitive, nonfunctional behavior. If children exhibited disruptive behaviors that greatly interfered with progress, physical punishment was used.

The control group, the other half, received an average of 10 h of ABA weekly as well as other treatments. Punishment was not used with the control group. So it was a comparison of intensity, punishment, and eclectic vs. ABA only. Children received intervention for two or more years and treatment occurred across environments: home, school, and the clinic.

At the end of treatment, all the children were independently evaluated. The outcome criteria of the three groups were based upon IQ, school placement, and diagnosis (Fig. 2.12).

OUTCOME CRITERIA

	"POOR"	"FAIR"	"BEST"
IQ	Profound-Severe	Moderate-Mild	Normal Range
School Placement	Classroom for Autistic Disorder	Special Education Other than Autistic Disorder	General Education WITHOUT Supports
Diagnosis	Autistic Disorder	Diagnosis Other Than Autistic Disorder	Indistinguishable

Fig. 2.12 Outcome Criteria from Lovaas (1987) intensive behavioral treatment study

Children whose IQs were in the profound and severe range and/or were in classrooms for autistic disorder and/or still presented with a diagnosis of autism were classified in the "poor group" at follow-up. Children who had IQs in the moderate to mild range and/or were placed in special education other than classrooms for autistic disorder (primarily communication disorder classrooms) and/or presented with a diagnosis other than autism (usually a communication disorder diagnosis) were classified to be in the "fair" outcome group. To be in the best outcome group meant IQs were in the normal range, they were in general education classrooms without supports, and they were indistinguishable. That is they did not present with the behaviors or characteristics diagnostic of autism.

These were the results for the children who received an average of 40 h a week of ABA only and received punishment (Fig. 2.13):

Two children were classified as having "poor" outcomes, eight in the "fair" outcome group, and nine achieved "best" outcomes. In terms of IQ change, the two children in the "poor" group lost an average of 15 IQ points, not surprising given the tests evaluated more abstract concepts. Those children in the "fair" outcome group had a gain of 11 IQ points and the children who were in the "best" outcome group had an average gain of 38 points.

Let us compare it to the control group who received an average of 10 h weekly of ABA, did not receive punishment, and received a variety of treatments including limited ABA (Fig. 2.14).

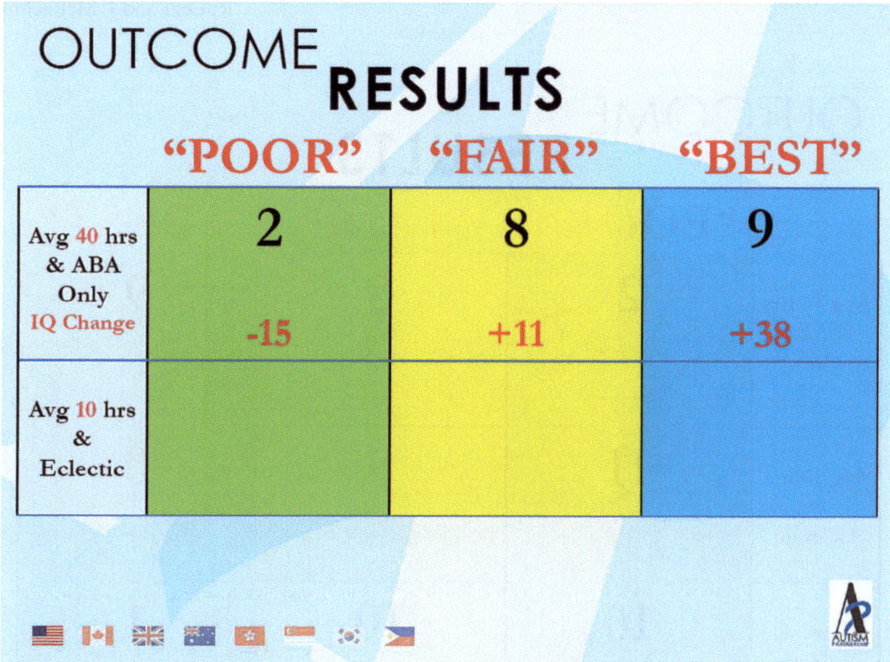

Fig. 2.13 Treatment Outcome for Intensive Treatment Group

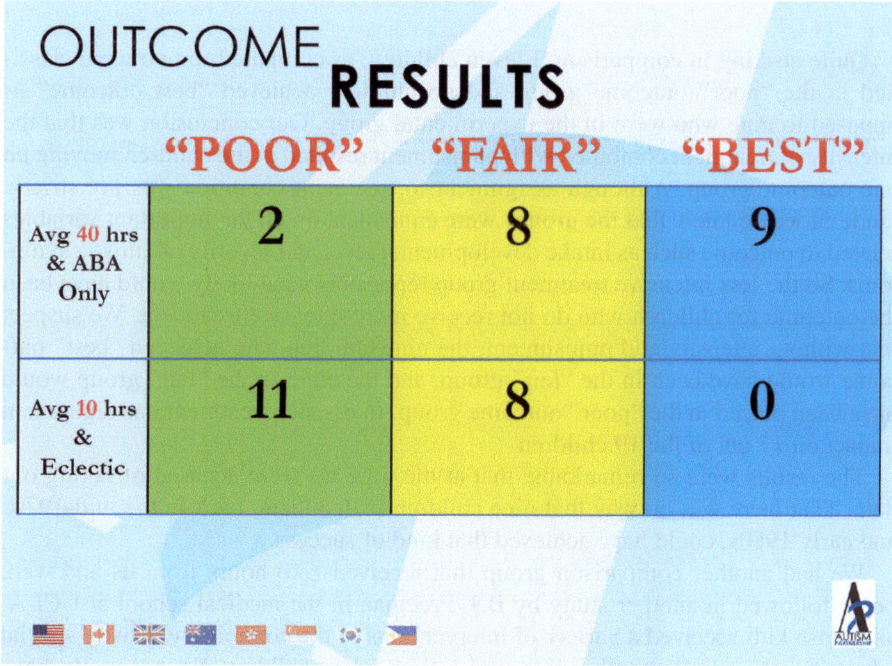

Fig. 2.14 Comparison Between Intensive Treatment vs Comparison Group 1

OUTCOME RESULTS

	"POOR"	"FAIR"	"BEST"
Avg 40 hrs & ABA Only	2	8	9
Avg 10 hrs & Eclectic	11	8	0
0 hrs & Eclectic	10	10	1

Fig. 2.15 Outcome for Comparison Group 2

Quite striking in comparison. Eleven children, as compared to two were classified in the "poor" outcome group and no children achieved "best outcome" as opposed to nine who were in the experimental group. Our conclusion was that the intensity of treatment combined with punishment resulted in the children moving up one outcome group. Although assignment to treatment condition was not strictly random, we do know that the groups were equivalent on all the important variables related to outcome such as intake developmental level and severity of autistic symptoms. So the less intensive treatment group represents what likely would have been the outcome for children who do not receive more intensive treatment. We suspect that without intensity and punishment, the nine children who achieved "best" outcome would have been in the "fair" group, and the eight in the "fair" group would have been placed in the "poor" outcome group. In essence treatment had significant impact on 17 out of the 19 children.

The results were so remarkable that at the time we were accused of faking our data. That there was no way that nine children with autism, back in the mid-1970s and early 1980s, could have achieved that kind of success.

We had another comparison group that received zero hours from us and were being followed in another study by B.J. Freeman in the medical school at UCLA, and those kids received a variety of interventions in the community, mostly special education classes. Remember this was a time when children did not really have access to ABA treatment and most people were anti-ABA. Here are the results for that comparison group (Fig. 2.15).

The results for the group that did not receive ABA are very comparable to the group who received less intensive ABA treatment, leading us to suspect that receiving 10 h of treatment weekly is not much better than zero hours of treatment.

Let me show you videos of children representative of the two groups, the "fair" and the "best" outcome group. This first clip is representative of a child that achieved "fair" outcome.

VIDEO CLIP #3: http://www.autismpartnership.com/post/video-links-lovaas-model

Next is a child that was in the best outcome group.

VIDEO CLIP #4: http://www.autismpartnership.com/post/video-links-lovaas-model

Indeed, he did go to college, he got his bachelor's and master's degrees, and he did drink the booze. He has a good group of friends and he has a high quality of life. And he was not unique. There were eight other children who had very similar outcomes to him as represented in the data.

The study was important to us for many reasons. One, it greatly changed our expectations. We came to fully believe that children with autism had amazing potential. Of course, it took a great deal of work. It raised the bar for us, in terms of our expectations, and we have even higher expectations today.

Common Myths and Misinterpretations

There are a tremendous number of myths and misinterpretations of the Young Autism Project (Leaf & McEachin, 2008). That is why I have been so obsessed. I want to take this opportunity to clarify the misinformation:

- *All children received a minimum of 40 h a week.* Not true whatsoever; it was an average of 40 h. It ranged from 18 to 60 h. The two children who were eventually placed in the "poor" outcome group received the most hours.
- *We only treated high-functioning children* (Schopler, Short, & Mesibov, 1989). After all if we did not fake the data how else could we have achieved such results? So we must have just treated high-functioning children. But remember the treatment occurred in the 1970s. Children who were "high functioning" would not have received a diagnosis of autism at that time. Also, the functioning levels were comparable in the two groups, so if it was not the treatment that made the difference, the less intensive treatment group should have done just as well.
- *Intervention was exclusively one to one.* One to one was certainly critical. It was the starting point of treatment. But as soon as possible we wanted children to be able to learn in small and then large groups. We needed to get them into school by the time they were five, so that they would be able to be in general education classrooms by First grade at the latest. We strongly believed in intervention being conducted in groups.
- *The treatment was punitive.* Although most of the children did receive physical punishment when they exhibited severe interfering behaviors, they always received far more reinforcement than punishment. And toward the end of the project we were no longer using physical punishment.

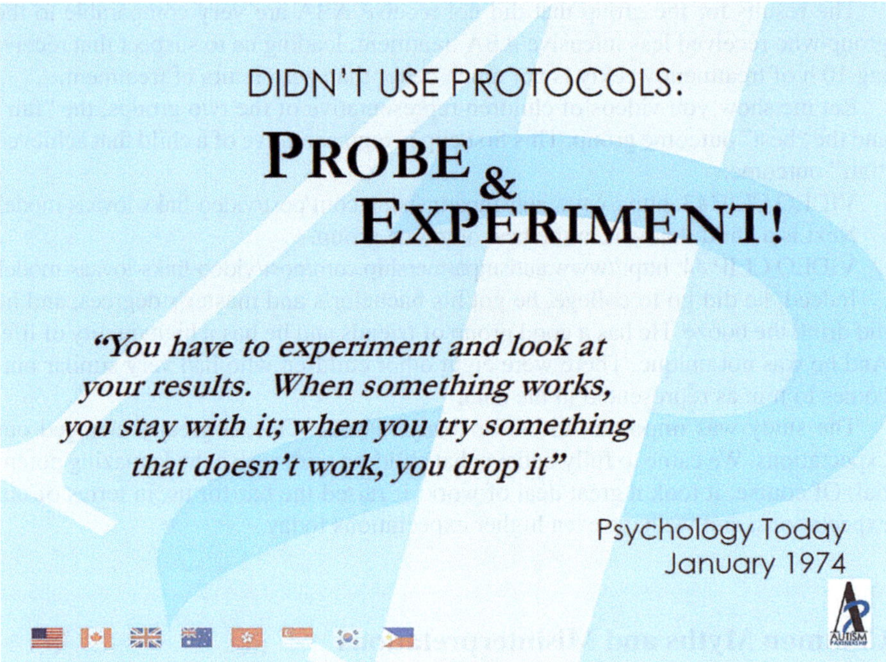

Fig. 2.16 Lovaas' view on protocols

- *Intervention was rigid and protocol driven* (Lipsker, Leaf, & Desio, 1978). Let me assure you, it was not rigid whatsoever. You saw the film from 50 years ago. It was not rigid back then and was not rigid during our generation either. And we were certainly not protocol driven. In fact, Ivar did not believe in protocols. He wanted us to be innovative, creative, and always changing. He wanted us to probe and of course evaluate if what we were doing was effective. If it was not effective then we would change the program. "Do not adhere to protocols!" (Chance & Lovaas, 1974) Similar to an outstanding cook, you may use a recipe as a guide but be creative and improvise as you deem necessary. With the children in the study we had a structure, a plan, but were always willing, encouraged and expected to change so as to meet the needs of our children. Individualization was critical and rigid protocols were antithetical to responding to the unique and ever changing needs of the child (Fig. 2.16).
- *The results are not replicable*. That is probably the number one criticism of the "Lovaas Model"! Indeed, there have been no studies that have achieved the same results. But, was that because we faked the data, or because we hand-selected clients, or that we only treated high-functioning children? I assure you, none of those accusations are true. I strongly believe the results have not been replicated because no one has followed, or perhaps could follow, what was done at UCLA. Let me suggest several factors that make it difficult, if not impossible to replicate the results.

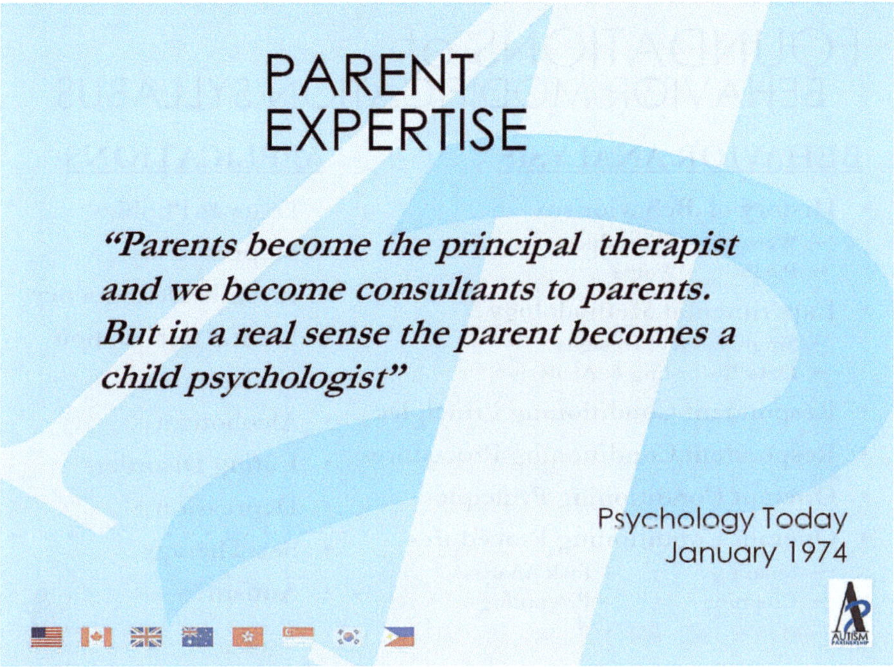

Fig. 2.17 Lovaas' view on parents' role

- One has to do with the use of physical punishment. Physical punishment was an important component of the treatment package and there are some things that today are much harder to achieve without the use of strong negative consequences, such as competing with the reinforcing power of self-stimulatory behavior. We stopped using physical punishment, not because it was ineffective; it was incredibly effective. We stopped it because it was not politically correct (Hayes & McCurry, 1990; Maurer, 1983). And today, it is highly unlikely that physical punishment will be used in treatment, at least not in this country. However, the good thing is that it forced us become more creative and more effective in the use of positive reinforcement.
- Parent expertise was absolutely essential. Based upon Ivar's original outcome study in 1973 (Lovaas et al., 1973) a central emphasis was developing parent expertise. Consequently one of the criteria to participate in the study was that one of the parents had to quit his/her job to be available as a full-time therapist. Our parents were so good at treatment that they helped train our staff. They were so good that during quarter breaks when the undergraduate students were on vacation, our children continued to progress because the parents were doing the treatment. When we implemented a new program, parents would sit down and pilot the program. Ivar commented that we were consultants to the parents; they were their child's psychologists. And indeed that is how it was (Fig. 2.17).

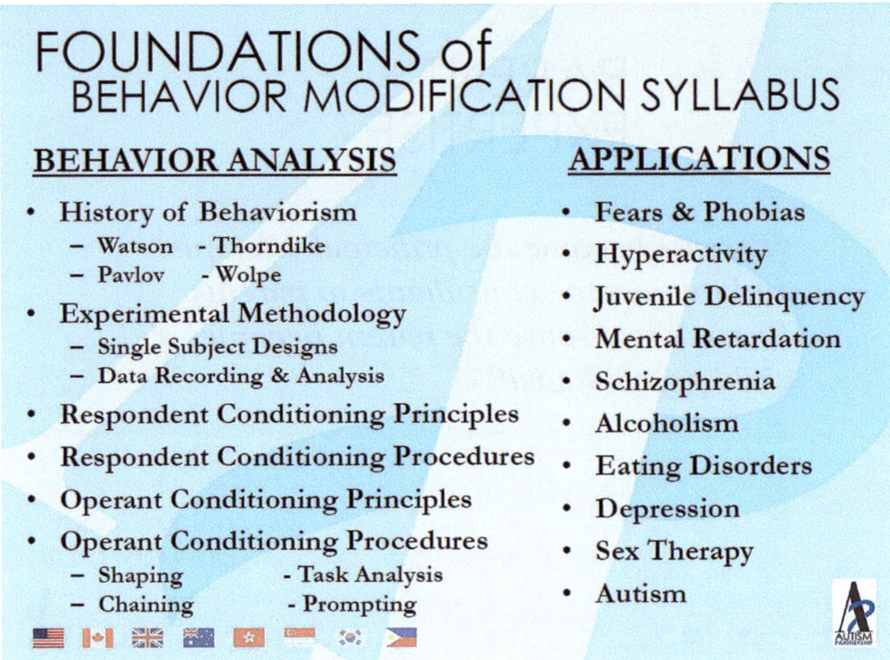

Fig. 2.18 UCLA Course Syllabus

– Another factor which makes replication difficult if not impossible was the level of staff expertise. Ivar was absolutely obsessed, possessed, about staff expertise. He recognized that children's outcomes were directly related to staff expertise. Training started in that Foundations of Behavior Modification class (Fig. 2.18).
– We were taught about the foundations of ABA, the importance of our founding ancestors and about the heart of ABA. We were taught that ABA grew from innovation and the pioneers being willing to be creative and take risks in order to help. We learned about utilizing the full range of behavioral treatment, not just operant techniques, but respondent as well.
– The class was divided into two segments. The first part focused on behavior analysis in which we learned the history of behaviorism, experimental methodology, respondent principles and procedures, and operant as well. The second half of the class turned toward the application of behavior analysis, the applied aspect across numerous populations. Autism was just one part of it.
– Comprehensive training and supervision was provided by Ivar's graduate students. Ivar was a believer that his graduate students needed to have a firm foundation in all of psychology, not just behaviorism. In fact, in graduate school, we rarely took a class in ABA. We learned about other schools of psychology because Ivar was a believer that we needed to have "insight." We needed to have clinical skills. We needed to be able to work with parents and professionals with sensitivity. Critical thinking was a huge emphasis. Not following set protocols

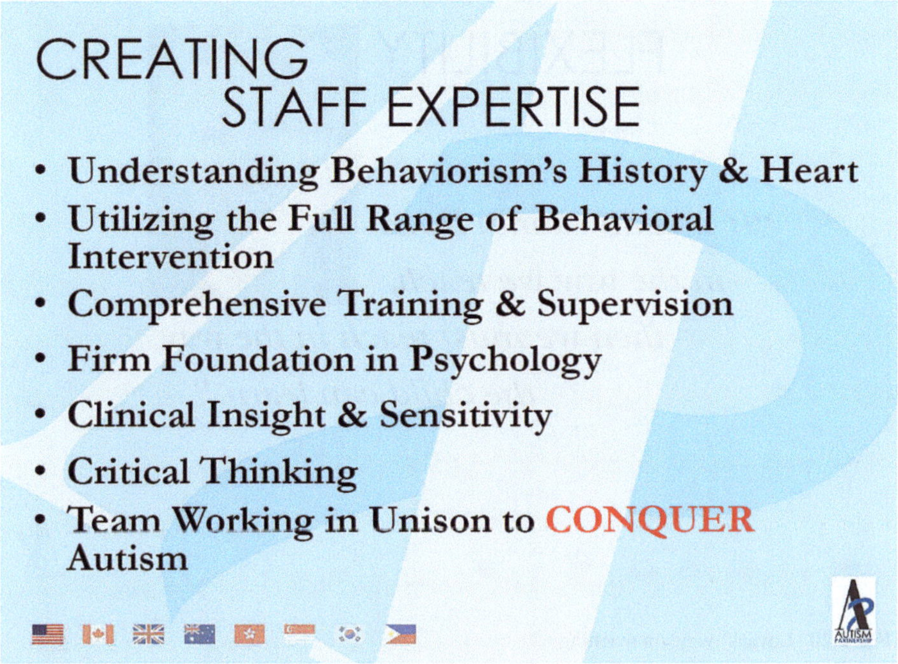

Fig. 2.19 UCLA YAP approach to staff development

meant we have to continually analyze and evaluate our work. Perhaps Ivar's biggest contribution to all the generations was that he created tremendous team unity. It is not surprising that 40 years later many of us are still working together. And this was true of most of the generations. He created teams that fully believed that we would conquer autism (Fig. 2.19).

- Ivar was always extremely concerned about professionals not having the proper expertise in ABA and the damage it would create for children, families, and the field. In 2002, Ivar shared his concern.
- VIDEO CLIP #5: http://www.autismpartnership.com/post/video-links-lovaas-model
  - Replicability is extremely difficult since this is an extremely complex model of intervention. The approach was flexible as I have already discussed and because of that it is very difficult to operationalize and certainly could not be distilled into a treatment manual. No protocols. Flexibility was absolutely essential (Lipsker et al., 1978). Ivar was often quoted as saying, "if children can't learn in the way we teach, then we must teach in a way they can learn" (Fig. 2.20).
- We needed to be flexible. And we needed to be critical thinkers. In preparing for this presentation, I uncovered a manual we wrote in 1978 (Lipsker et al., 1978). On one page the word "flexible" appeared seven times (Fig. 2.21).

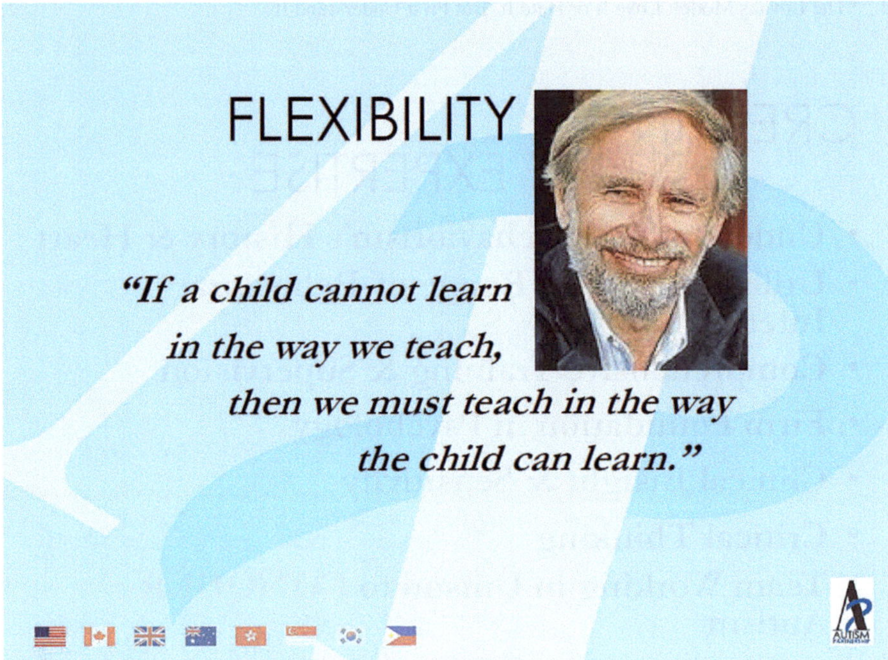

Fig. 2.20 Lovaas' view on teaching

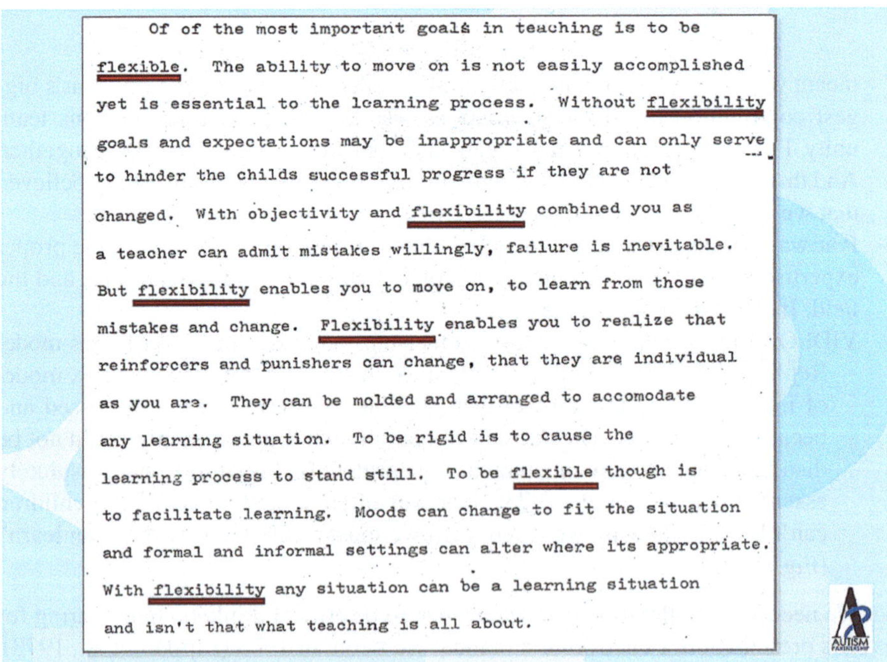

Of of the most important goals in teaching is to be flexible. The ability to move on is not easily accomplished yet is essential to the learning process. Without flexibility goals and expectations may be inappropriate and can only serve to hinder the childs successful progress if they are not changed. With objectivity and flexibility combined you as a teacher can admit mistakes willingly, failure is inevitable. But flexibility enables you to move on, to learn from those mistakes and change. Flexibility enables you to realize that reinforcers and punishers can change, that they are individual as you are. They can be molded and arranged to accomodate any learning situation. To be rigid is to cause the learning process to stand still. To be flexible though is to facilitate learning. Moods can change to fit the situation and formal and informal settings can alter where its appropriate. With flexibility any situation can be a learning situation and isn't that what teaching is all about.

Fig. 2.21 Draft of teaching manual during YAP era

So, why is the Lovaas model so misinterpreted? Well, these are some possible reasons:

- Often people think of the Lovaas Model as being one of electric shock. Still today, professionals tell me they reject ABA because they do not believe in electric shock. They do not believe in slapping children's faces! Well neither do we. But that was over 50 years ago when it was the pioneering days of treating ASD (e.g., Lovaas, Schaeffer, & Simmons, 1965). If we are going to evaluate things based on 50 years ago, we would be in trouble. We most likely would not agree to bypass surgery if we observed heart surgery from 50 years ago.
- I think, perhaps, some of the misinterpretations have to do with the ***Me Book*** (Lovaas, 1981). A book that Ivar and colleagues wrote in the mid-1970s. That was already outdated by the time our generation left. In fact, we stopped using it before it was even published. Ivar saw the book as a book of basic recipes that required adaptation, innovation and analysis. Unfortunately, more than 30 years later people are still using the book as a strict protocol. Meanwhile, critics point to it as evidence of what a bad idea it is to do ABA therapy with children who have ASD.
- I think a great deal of the misinterpretation actually has to do with practitioners in the field that claim they are following the Lovaas model. But in fact they have an extremely narrow interpretation of the model:
  - For example, professionals believe they are following the model when they eliminate distractions (Green, 2001). In schools, children often work in distraction free classrooms: they work in cubicles or behind partitions with reduced noise and interruptions. Home therapy is often conducted exclusively in a therapy room.

- Well, in reality, Ivar thought we needed to work in the most natural setting possible. He wanted chaos. I remember one case where we sat on the floor, with the TV blaring, and the windows were open so the child could see other children playing outside. Ivar recognized we would not achieve generalization if we did not work in natural environments.
  - There is a false belief that our teaching style was extremely stilted and unnatural. The belief was that we issued one-word instructions, never varied our instructions and used the same tone of voice (Green, 2001). In essence we were robots! However, if we were robots we would not have produced natural language and generalization would not have occurred. Although we were systematic, we strived to be as natural and playful as possible.
  - One on one was certainly central but as I have shared, group work was also essential.
  - Many people think we exclusively used discrete trial teaching, called discrete trail "**training**" back then. Yes, we did rely upon DTT, but we also used other instructional formats as well. We used incidental teaching (Hart & Risley, 1975) and Mitch Taubman brought teaching interactions (Phillips, Phillips, Fixsen, & Wolf, 1974) back from Kansas as another instructional format.

- The Lovaas Model is often associated with the use of food reinforcement and more specifically the use of m&m's. Yes, we often **initially** used food, but we quickly developed toys and activities to substitute for food. More important was using social engagement and developing relationships. Reinforcement development required creativity and not relying on protocols but using what we now call clinical judgment or in-the-moment assessments (Leaf, Kassardjian, et al., 2016; Leaf, Leaf, et al., 2015, 2016; Leaf, Oppenheim-Leaf, et al., 2015; Soluaga, Leaf, Taubman, McEachin, & Leaf, 2008). I will more fully discus "clinical judgment" when I talk about our work at Autism Partnership.
- As discussed previously, perhaps the biggest misinterpretation was that we followed strict protocols. However, it simply would not have addressed the children's unique needs. It certainly would have been easier to train staff if we had used a set recipe and would have been easier for staff to implement because they would not have to think and adjust. But following strict protocols was not the Lovaas model in our generation and not in previous generations either.

• I think perhaps some of the misinterpretation of the Lovaas Model has to do with Ivar being a controversial figure. He simply loved controversy. One night he was at a dinner with 12 psychiatrists. He stood up, held up a bowl of salad, and then proclaimed that there were more brains in this salad than in the room and then he walked out. That does not get you fans for your approach. In 2004, he made a statement if he had gotten Hitler at the age of four or five he could have made him be a nicer person, maybe even a humanitarian (Ito, 2004) (Fig. 2.22).

• By the way, is not this John B. Watson reincarnated? Ivar was controversial for sure. Unfortunately, this may have contributed to disdain of Ivar's work and led to misunderstanding of the work done at UCLA.

VIDEO CLIP #6: http://www.autismpartnership.com/post/video-links-lovaas-model
By the way, that is Don Baer who was speaking in the video clip (Baer, 2002).

Conceptual Basis of the YAP Approach

Now, I am going to share our approach at Autism Partnership. Clearly our roots are grounded from the UCLA Young Autism Project. But prior to founding Autism Partnership in 1994, we had a variety of other experiences (Fig. 2.23).

In the late 1970s, Ivar and I founded Behavior Therapy and Learning Center. The focus of the Center was to provide training and support to parents who had children not only with Autism but also all disabilities. In the early 1980s, we entered into the adult world. For 15 years we provided comprehensive treatment in residential and vocational settings to clients with a variety of disabilities. This was during the days of deinstitutionalization. We were taking adults with severe and persistent behavior problems out of state hospitals and placing them into the community. We learned

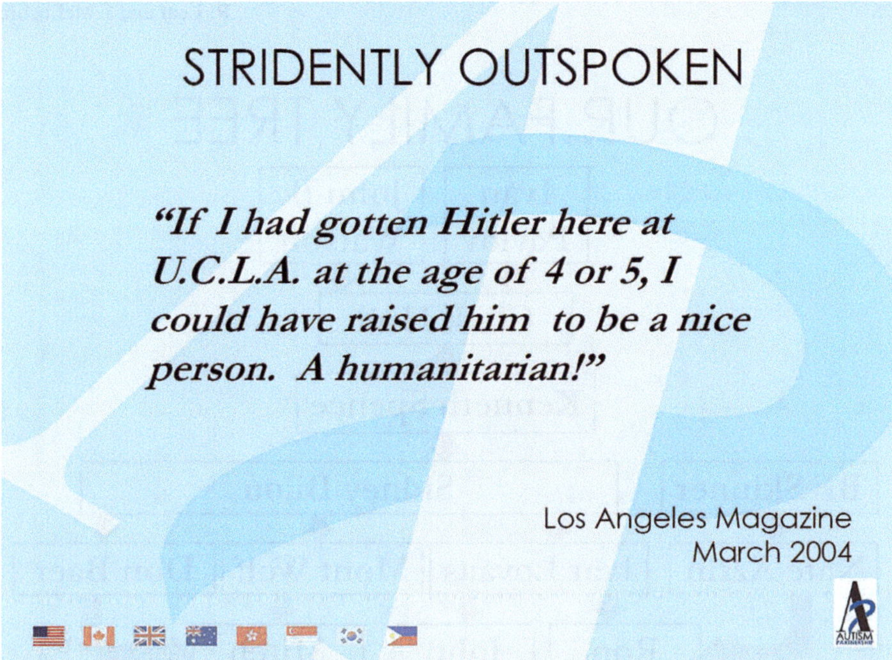

Fig. 2.22 Example of Lovaas' unbridled retoric.

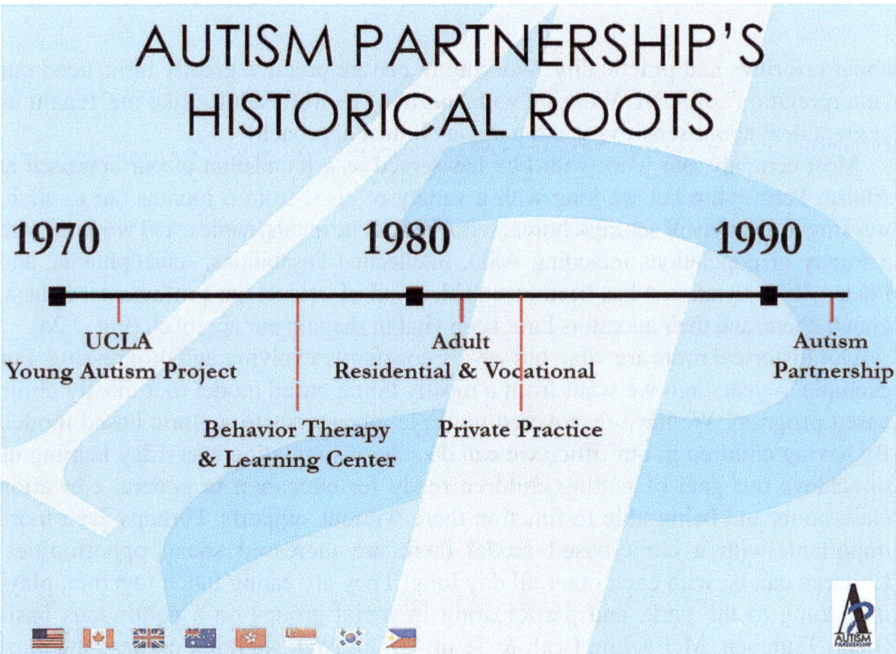

Fig. 2.23 Autism Partnership's Historical Roots

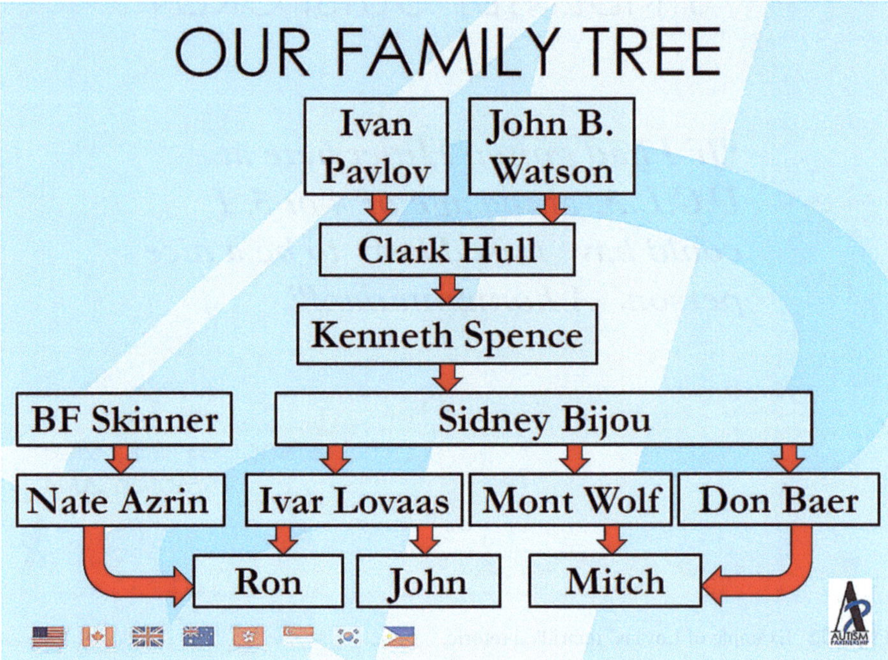

Fig. 2.24 Autism Partnership Family Tree

about priorities and practicality. Working in private practice greatly influenced our "interpretation" of ABA. Working with "normal" neurotic adults, like me, taught us at great deal about sensitivity and using a clinical approach!

Most certainly, our work with Ivar has served as a foundation of our approach at Autism Partnership but working with a variety of ages, from 6 months old to adult, working in a variety of settings, home, schools, state hospitals, clinics, and working with a variety of populations including ASD, Intellectual Disabilities, schizophrenia, and Prader–Willi Syndrome has been invaluable. And of course, our professional fathers, grandfathers, and their ancestors have been vital in shaping our approach (Fig. 2.24).

Our historical roots are vital, but we are constantly evolving and progressing. For example, 5 years ago we went from a mostly home based model to a mostly clinic based program. We have discovered multiple advantages to a clinic based model. By having children in our office we can do school simulation every day helping us to achieve our goal of getting children ready for education in general education classrooms and being able to function there without supports. Perhaps even more important, with a clinic-based model there are increased social opportunities. Children can be with each other all day long. They are eating lunch together, playing, going to the park, and participating in social groups on a continuous basis (Leaf, Taubman, McEachin, Leaf, & Tsuji, 2011). And, we think perhaps the most important part of being a clinic-based model is that we are able to provide our staff with training, supervision and support on a continuous basis.

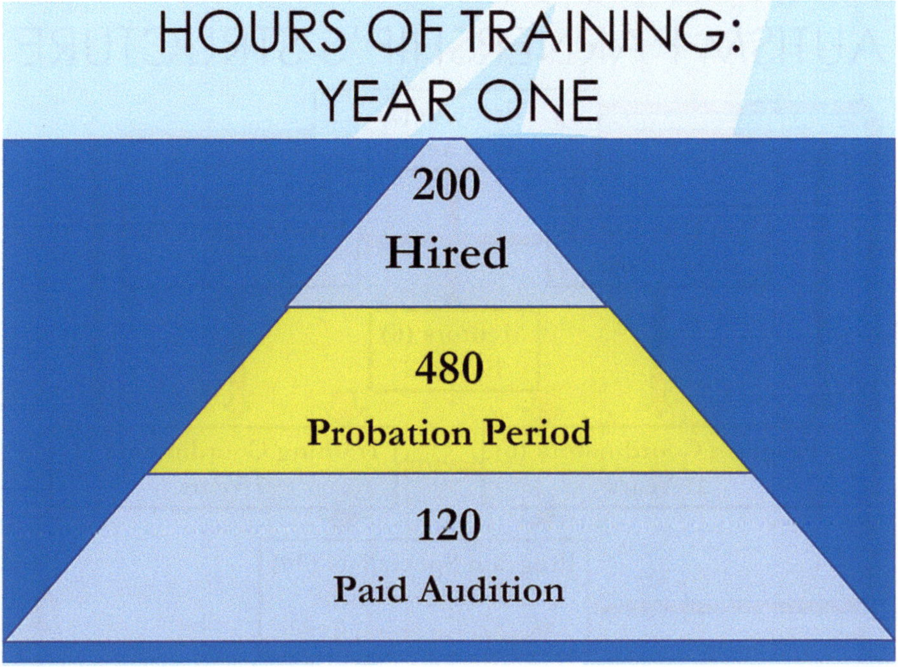
HOURS OF TRAINING:
YEAR ONE
200
Hired
480
Probation Period
120
Paid Audition

Fig. 2.25 Autism Partnership Family Tree

Staff Training and Expertise

We are committed to extensive staff development and training, and it starts with the recruiting process. We typically get 100 resumes a week. Out of those 100, we reject 90 and interview only 10. Based on the first interview, we typically ask five to return for a second interview. From those five, we generally invite three applicants to participate in a paid audition for up to 1 month. During this time, we provide them training in the basics of ABA and they observe our work and interact with the children. They get to know us, we get to know them and we are better able to decide if we think it is a good fit. Typically, two applicants make it through the process. At this point they have already received 120 h of training. But now the real training begins! (Fig. 2.25).

Before working independently, a new staff member receives 480 h of training which includes discussions, reading, observations, and working with children under the guidance of supervisors and staff trainers. In order for staff to gain all the skills necessary to make in-the-moment assessments, we feel such training is a critical investment. They have got to be critical thinkers, they have to constantly analyze what is happening, and we feel it will only occur with extensive and comprehensive training. In the book, *Outliers* the author suggested that it takes 10,000 h to become an expert. When it comes to providing quality ABA, we think actually think that is

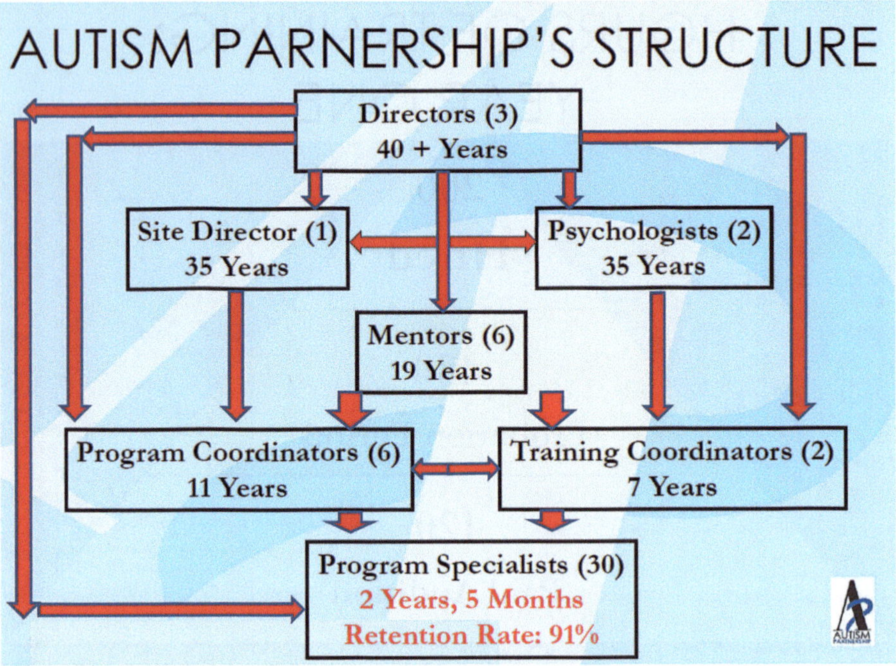

Fig. 2.26 Autism Partnership Organizational Structure

an underestimate. We have found for staff to become extremely skilled it is usually a 5 to 10 year process.

Our structure is very similar to what we had at UCLA. We also use a tiered approach. The advanced clinical staff, the old people, have been together since the mid-1970s. Then we have got the newer staff, our mentors who have been part of AP for 19 years. The next level is our coordinators and supervisors. And then our direct line staff which have a retention rate of 91 % (for staff who complete the training process) (Fig. 2.26).

Role of Parents

Parent buy-in and expertise is essential. When we screen parents we share with them our expectations. We do not want them to become therapists, as we did at UCLA. We want parents to be Mommy and Daddy, not therapists. However, they must become extremely knowledgeable. It is essential that they fully understand, and are supportive of what we are doing. And perhaps most importantly that they embrace ABA and do not do alternative, nonevidence-based treatments (Leaf, Kassardjian, et al., 2016; Leaf, Leaf, et al., 2016). We want them to be able to work with their children on the weekends, not in formal therapy, but to generalize what we are doing.

Primary Procedural Components

These are our phases of intervention (Fig. 2.27).

Obviously every child is different and their treatment plans vary based upon their unique needs. Typically, however, we start off with reducing interfering behaviors. Acting out behaviors such as, aggression, noncompliance, tantrums, or passive behavior problems such as inattention or self-stimulation have to be significantly reduced. Whether it takes 1 day, 1 month, or 1 year we have to address these interfering behaviors in order to successfully teach communication, play, and social skills. Behavior change requires reactive strategies that immediately address the behaviors when they occur. More important are the proactive strategies that teach our children appropriate alternatives and that address the function of the interfering behaviors (Fig. 2.28).

Once interfering behaviors are decreasing, we then target "learning how to learn" skills (Leaf et al., 2011). At UCLA we recognized the importance of teaching children preparatory skills. Today, however we feel it is absolutely essential to teach children how to learn. We think it is taken for granted that children have these skills. However, if a child will not give back their reinforcer or return from breaks, it makes teaching very difficult. They have to learn how to pay attention. That does not mean eye contact, developed through "look at me" drills. Eye contact is just one

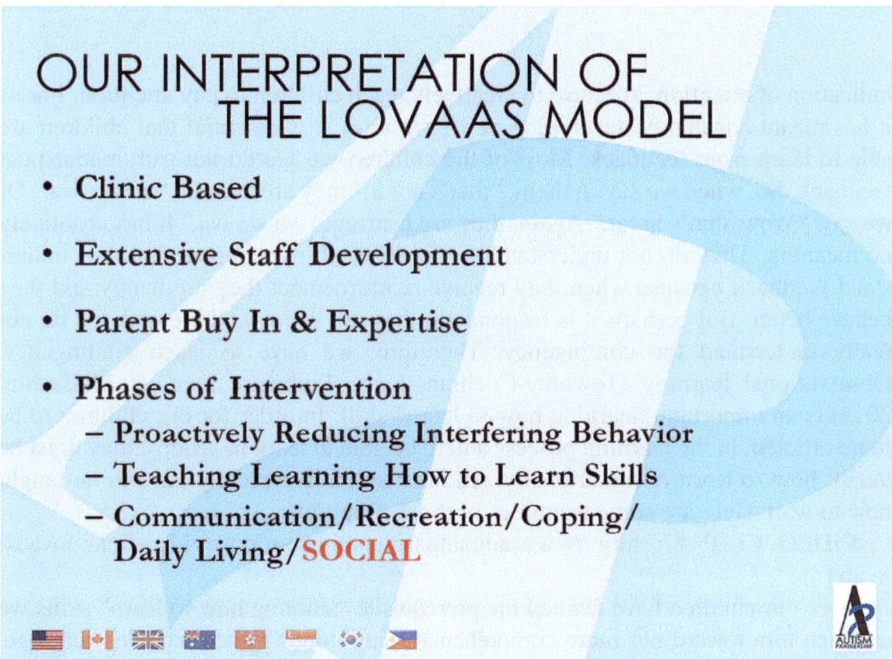

Fig. 2.27 Phases of intervention

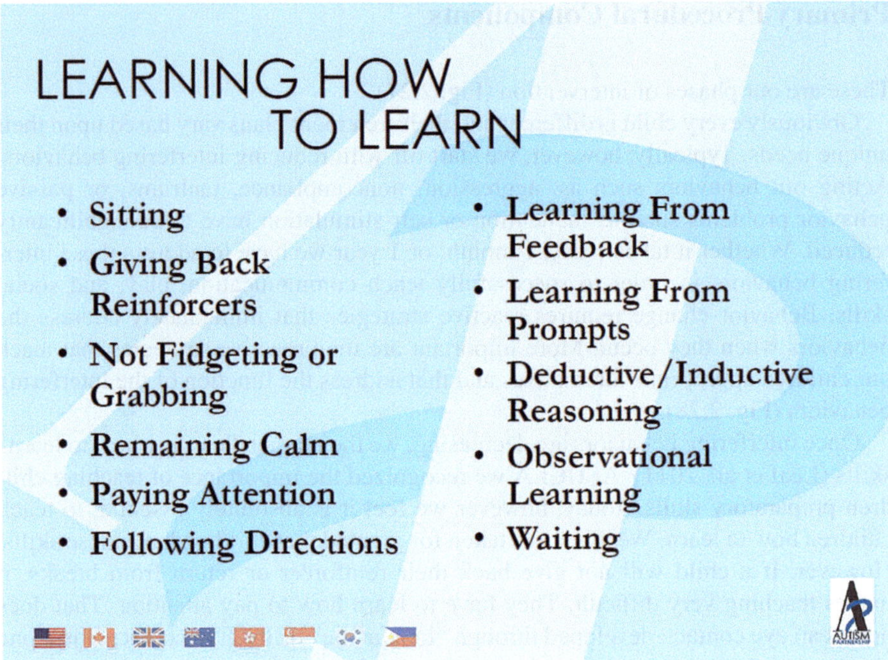

Fig. 2.28 Learning How to Learn

indication of attention. We have to creatively teach children to pay attention. For us it has meant constantly developing new programs. It is essential that children are able to learn from feedback. Most of the children we see do not truly understand feedback. So, when we say to them, "that's not it," they are hearing "wa wa wa." Or we say, "Wow, that's great." Again, they are hearing, "wa wa wa." It has absolutely no meaning. They do not understand the feedback. It may appear that they understand feedback because when they receive reinforcement they are happy and they behave better. But perhaps it is respondent; they are happy and pleased, but do not really understand the contingency. Therefore, we have to teach contingency. Observational learning (Townley-Cochran, Leaf, Taubman, Leaf, & McEachin, 2015) is an important "learning how to learn" skill. In order for our children to be more efficient in the learning process and to be able to learn in groups, they must be taught how to learn observationally. And our children typically have to be taught how to wait. Here are some examples of those programs:

VIDEO CLIP #7: http://www.autismpartnership.com/post/video-links-lovaas-model

Once our children have learned the prerequisite "learning how to learn" skills we can then turn toward our more comprehensive curriculum which includes language, social, play, self-help, and stress management—everything a child needs (Leaf & McEachin, 1999). We just do not just treat one aspect of the child, we treat the whole child.

Social is capitalized and in red because we want to emphasize that when teaching our children, social skills are paramount. When children learn social skills they can have meaningful friendships. When all is said and done a child learning to speak or mastering academics is not as important as developing meaningful friendships! Learning social skills simply leads to a higher quality of life, so this is our ultimate objective.

Selecting and Sequencing Goals

How do we make our decisions, how do we select our curriculum? Well, we do not use paper and pencil tests unless we are doing research. We are looking child by child, and there are multiple factors that help us decide what curriculum to use (Fig. 2.29).

These are just some of the factors that we consider: What behaviors are interfering with the learning process? What skill deficits do they have? We look at the chronological age as well as the developmental age of our clients. What skills would help increase their understanding of feedback? We are looking at what skills would be motivating for the child to learn. What would *he* want to learn? What excites

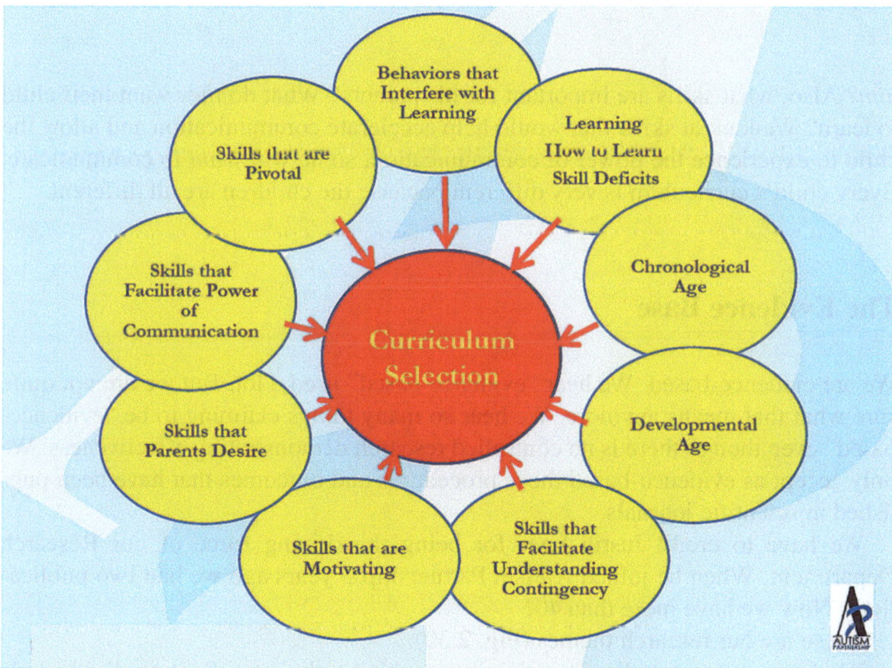

Fig. 2.29 Considerations in Selection of Curriculum

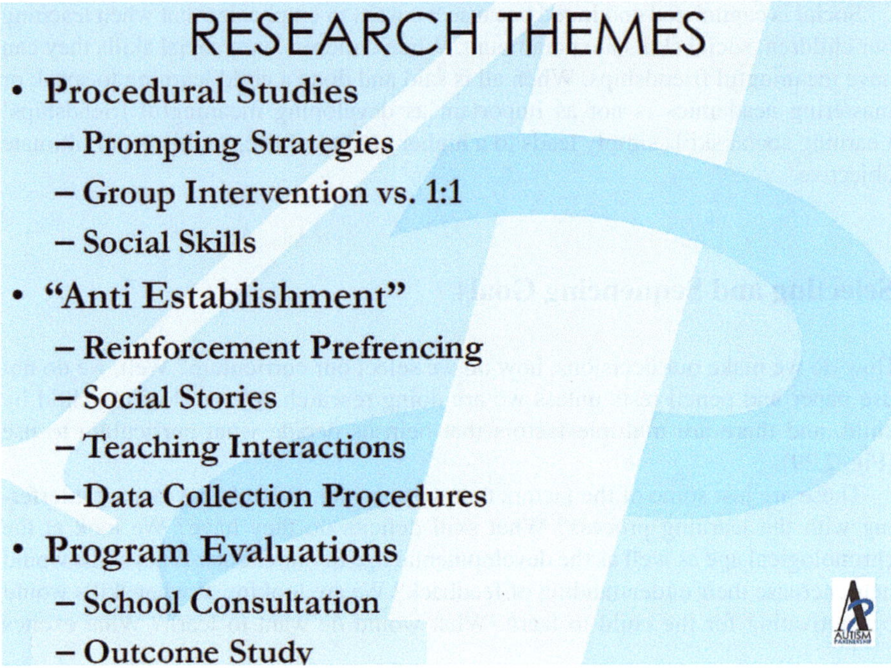
RESEARCH THEMES
• Procedural Studies
– Prompting Strategies
– Group Intervention vs. 1:1
– Social Skills
• "Anti Establishment"
– Reinforcement Prefrencing
– Social Stories
– Teaching Interactions
– Data Collection Procedures
• Program Evaluations
– School Consultation
– Outcome Study
AUTISM

Fig. 2.30 Autism Partnership research themes

him? Also, what skills are important for his parents? What do *they* want their child to learn? We look at skills that would help accelerate communication and allow the child to experience the power of communication, so he will *want* to communicate. Every child's curriculum is very different because the children are all different.

The Evidence Base

We are evidence-based. We hear "evidence-based" used a lot. But we are not quite sure what that means anymore. We hear so many things claiming to be "evidence-based" even though there is no controlled research demonstrating effectiveness. We only accept as evidence-based those procedures and outcomes that have been published in scientific journals.

We have to credit Justin Leaf for being the driving force of our Research Department. When he joined Autism Partnership 5 years ago we had two publications. Now we have more than 40!

These are our research themes (Fig. 2.30):

We do procedural studies investigating teaching techniques. Such studies include examining prompting strategies (Leaf, Leaf, Alcalay, et al., 2014; Leaf, Leaf,

Taubman, McEachin, & Delmolino, 2014; Soluaga et al., 2008) comparing errorless learning, versus "no, no, prompting" versus flexible prompt fading (Leaf, Sheldon, & Sherman, 2010). We have examined the effectiveness of group intervention as contrasted with 1:1 (Leaf et al., 2013). We have conducted studies examining various procedures to teach our children social skills (Leaf, Oppenheim-Leaf, et al., 2012; Leaf, Tsuji, et al., 2012).

We also do what we call "antiestablishment" studies. Looking at procedures that are widely used in ABA and examining if they are truly effective. We researched different data collection procedures (Taubman, Leaf, McEachin, Papovich, & Leaf, 2013). Many professionals consider continuous data collection to be the gold standard. But is it really necessary and are there disadvantages? Our study suggested that perhaps there are better alternatives. Recently, we examined reinforcer preference assessments (Leaf, Leaf, et al., 2015; Leaf, Oppenheim-Leaf, et al., 2015), once again considered the gold standard, to identify effective reinforcers. Our data indicate that it is not often necessary to do formal preference assessments and more importantly it significantly reduces trials of learning. Social Stories are often being used by BCBA's but are they really effective? Our research indicates that Teaching Interactions, developed decades ago at the University of Kansas are far more effective as a strategy. When examined carefully, Social Stories unless accompanied by other teaching strategies turn out to be largely ineffective (Kassardjian et al., 2014; Leaf, Leaf, et al., 2015; Leaf, Oppenheim-Leaf, et al., 2012, 2015; Leaf, Tsuji, et al., 2012).

In 2011, we did a program evaluation looking at what we did, not an experimental study but rather a descriptive study (Leaf et al., 2011). We wanted to evaluate the effectiveness of our approach across four of our offices (US, Hong Kong, UK, and Australia). We used outcome criteria that were similar to what we used at UCLA (Fig. 2.31).

Forty-five out of sixty-four children achieved what we considered "best outcome."

Clinical Judgment: In the Moment Assessment

Clinical judgment is perhaps that most important aspect of our approach at Autism Partnership (Leaf, Kassardjian, et al., 2016; Leaf, Leaf, et al., 2016). We are continuously making in-the-moment assessments, meaning we are analyzing second-by-second what to do, not being protocol driven. Not being a slave to the recipe, but altering the recipe continuously.

Why clinical judgment? Well, because it is not black and white. And our children do not read the protocols. Why clinical judgment? Stokes & Baer's, 1977 article, one of my favorite articles in ABA, discussed how to achieve generalization. What they suggested is the same thing we mean when we say clinical judgment, continuously altering intervention. Why clinical judgment? Because Ivar taught us that is was an essential part of effective treatment. And the results we get are better when interventionists use their brain, than when they mindlessly follow protocol.

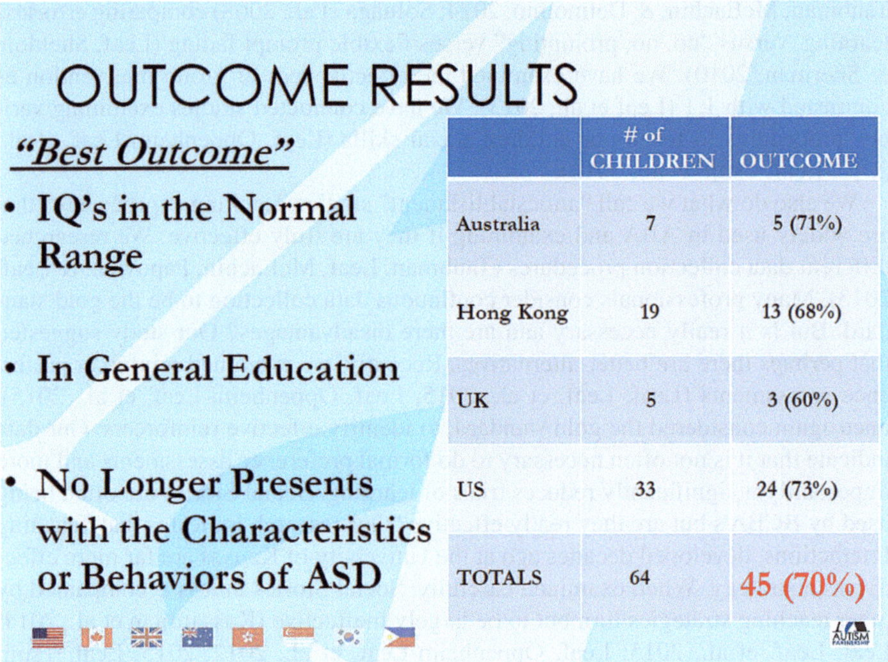

Fig. 2.31 Outcome classification for children receiving treatment at Autism Partnership

These are just some examples of in-the-moment assessments we are making (Fig. 2.32):

Complexity of teacher's language: Should our language be simple? Or should it be complex? Or in between? In reality, it often changes second by second and certainly child by child. Should the therapist select the reinforcers or the child? Or should we just probe and analyze the effect on the child's behavior and performance? Prompting strategies: Which one should we use? Well in reality there is no really one correct strategy. There are several effective prompting strategies and it changes moment by moment. What should be the targets? Which data collection procedure? In reality we do not often need to be collecting trial-by-trial data. We are killing too many trees! We can often take representative samples of data or simply do estimations and obtain valid summaries. We have to take data, but we have to first decide which collection procedure is optimal and reevaluate based upon clinical judgment (Fig. 2.33).

These are just some of the factors that we need to consider when making decisions–that is, the factors that influence our in-the-moment assessments, our "clinical judgment." Is the behavior operant or respondent? Because if it is respondent we should react very differently. What are the interfering behaviors? What is the function of behaviors? And there are certainly more than four possible functions of behavior. The current attentiveness of the child is essential in the decision-making process.

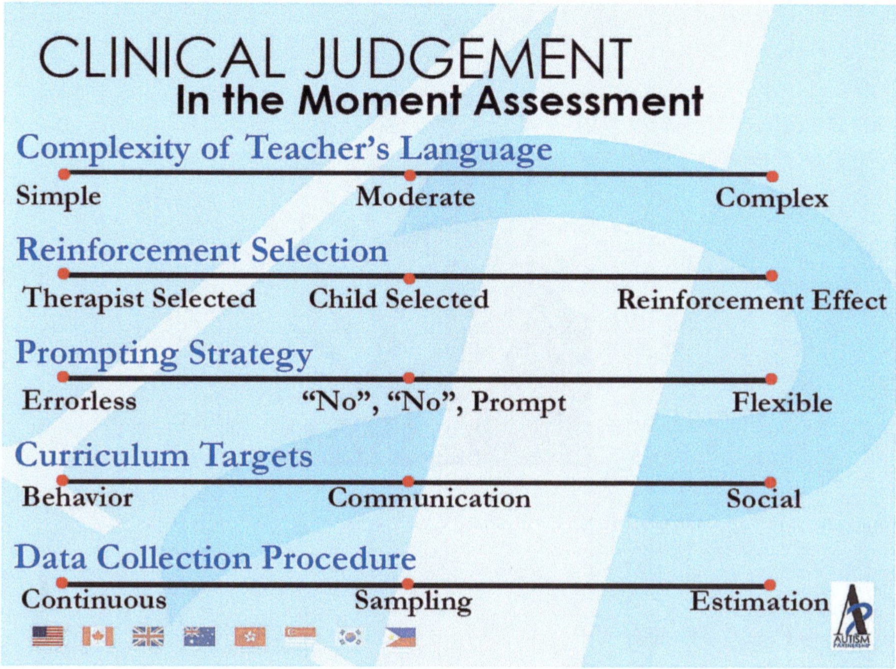

Fig. 2.32 In-the-moment decision making by interventionists

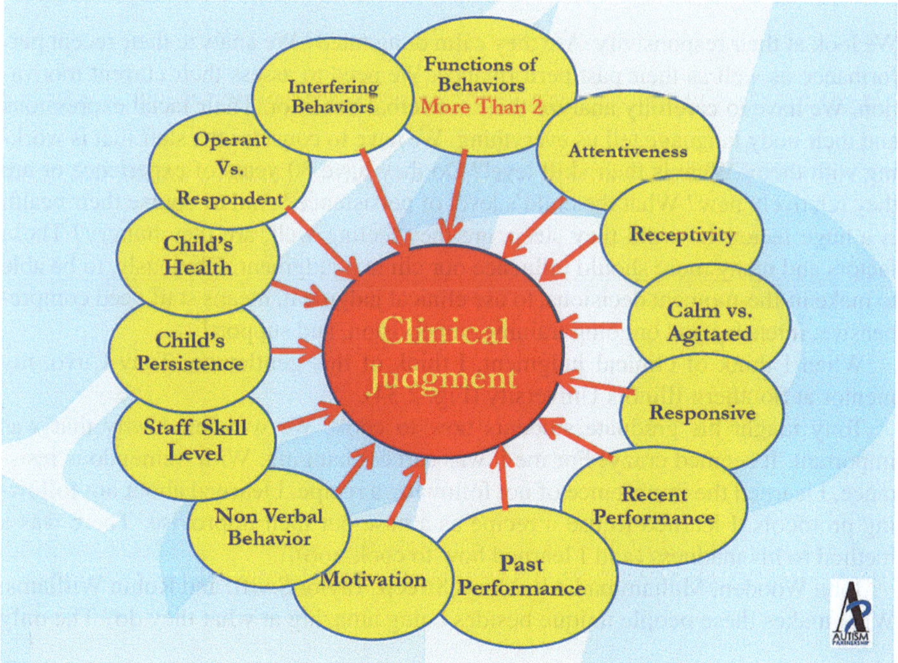

Fig. 2.33 Considerations that Factor into Clinical Judgment

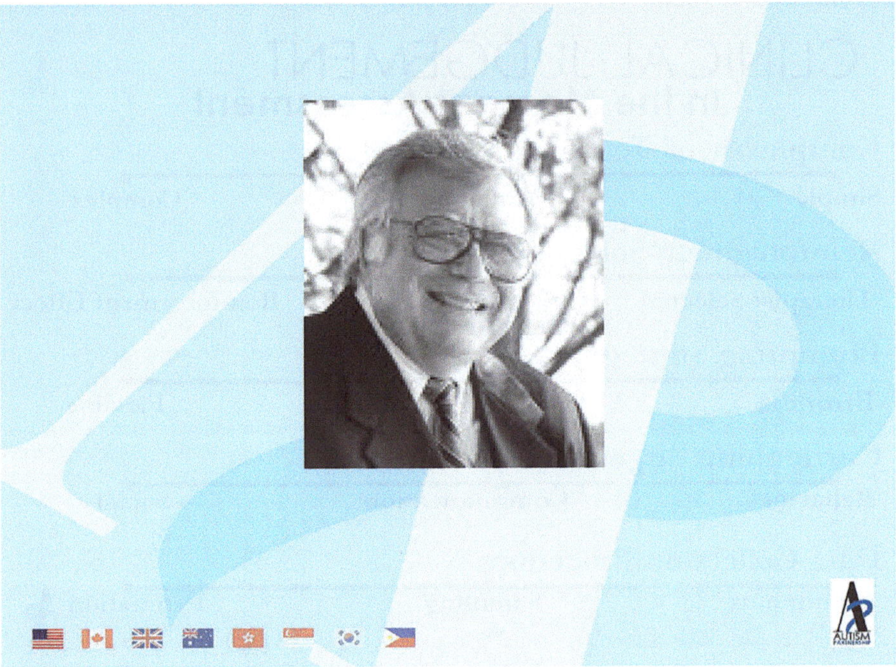

Fig. 2.34 Anthony Cuvo, mentor and chef

We look at their responsivity. Are they calm or agitated? We analyze their recent performance as well as their past performance. We need to assess their current motivation. We have to carefully analyze their nonverbal behavior. Their facial expressions and their body language tell us everything. We have to consider the staff that is working with them. What is their skill level? Do they have 30 years of experience or are they relatively new? What the child's level of persistence? And of course their health is a huge factor: how did they sleep, are they feeling well, are they hungry? These factors and many more should influence our clinical judgment. Obviously, to be able to make in-the-moment decisions, to use clinical judgment, means staff need comprehensive, intensive and ongoing training, supervision, and support!

When I think of clinical judgment, I think of this gentleman, Tony Cuvo, my mentor at Southern Illinois University (Fig. 2.34).

Tony taught his graduate students how to cook. We wondered why that was important. It seemed crazy! For me it was career changing. With tremendous resistance, I learned the importance of not following a recipe, I learned about not following protocols. I learned to use a recipe as a base but then improvise. There was a method to his madness (and I learned how to cook, too).

John Wooden, Muhammad Ali, Meryl Streep, Taylor Swift, and Robin Williams. What makes these people unique besides being amazing at what they do? The only

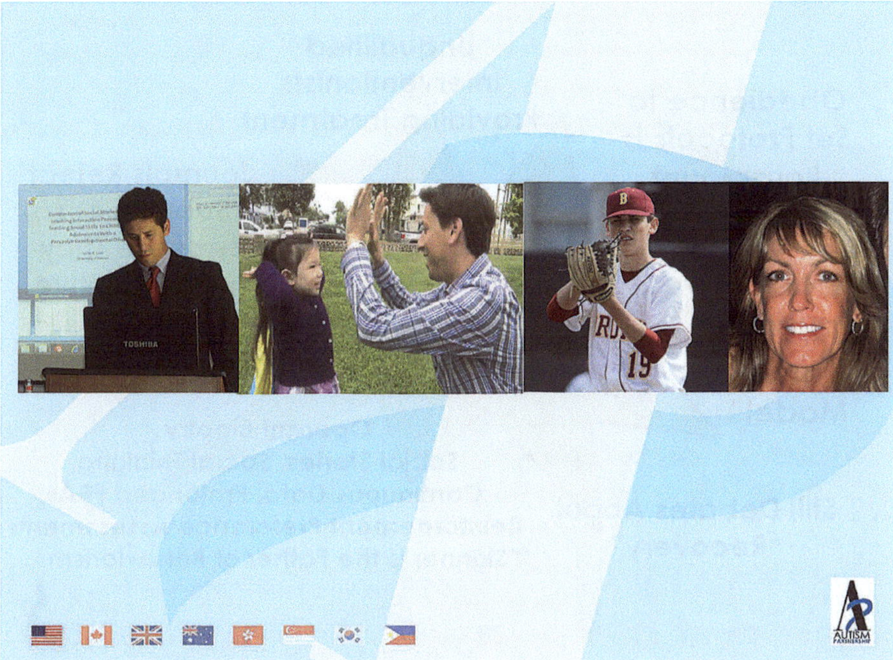

Fig. 2.35 Clinical judgment in all walks of life

one you may not know is John Wooden who I believe is the greatest coach of any sport! What makes them unique? They all used clinical judgment. Muhammad Ali, the best fight ever, he often fought with no fight plan, constantly changing his strategy based upon his clinical judgment. Robin Williams, obviously brilliant, clinical judgment.

Nate Azrin, Don Baer, Jim Sherman, Todd Risley, Mont Wolf, and Ted Ayllon—these are some of my heroes in the ABA world; they were the heart of ABA. They all used clinical judgment. They were all creative. They were all innovative. They did not follow protocols. That is the essence of ABA, just conquering the disorder, being brilliant. Ted Ayllon, developing the token economy, had no game plan, no protocol; he just probed and came up with it.

My family exudes clinical judgment. My son, Justin is a brilliant researcher because he uses clinical judgment. My middle son Jeremy is a wonderful therapist, he uses clinical judgment. My youngest son Cole is a pitcher and he uses clinical judgment, deciding what pitch to throw, what arm angle to use. My wife, Jamie is a brilliant therapist, she uses clinical judgment. She reads body language and facial expressions and how couples look at each other. This is what it takes to be outstanding. This is what it takes to make differences (Fig. 2.35).

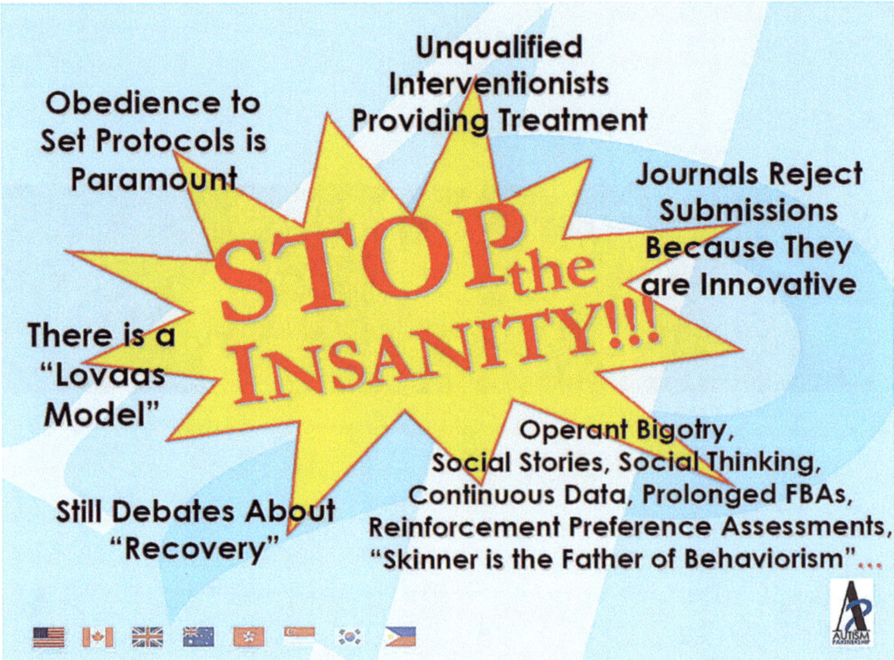

Fig. 2.36 Let's stop the insanity

Conclusion

Similar to Ivar we too are controversial, perhaps thought provoking. Maybe that is what it takes to stop the insanity in the world of ABA. Here is what I mean by insanity (Fig. 2.36):

We have actually had articles rejected because they are innovative. Journals have actually rejected articles because there has not been any research that had shown a new procedure to be effective! Of course there is none, we are doing the research. Operant bigotry: I am sad that in graduate school these days, people are not learning about respondent conditioning. And although respondent conditioning is a major factor in our children's behaviors it is being neglected. And Behaviorists are using Social Stories and Social Thinking! (Leaf, Kassardjian, et al., 2016; Leaf, Leaf, et al., 2016)! Really? Where is the research for those approaches? It is sad, it is tragic. Continuous data—where is the evidence that we need continuous data? Prolonged FBAs: for gosh sakes, most FBAs can be done in minutes. Of course, there are times a more extensive FBA is necessary but often not. And we are often endangering children with prolonged FBAs. Preference assessments? Do not get me started. And there are still debates about recovery, for God sakes. I do not get it! There is research, independent research, showing recovery does happen. Maybe recovery is not a good term and yes, we need to be careful about promoting recovery

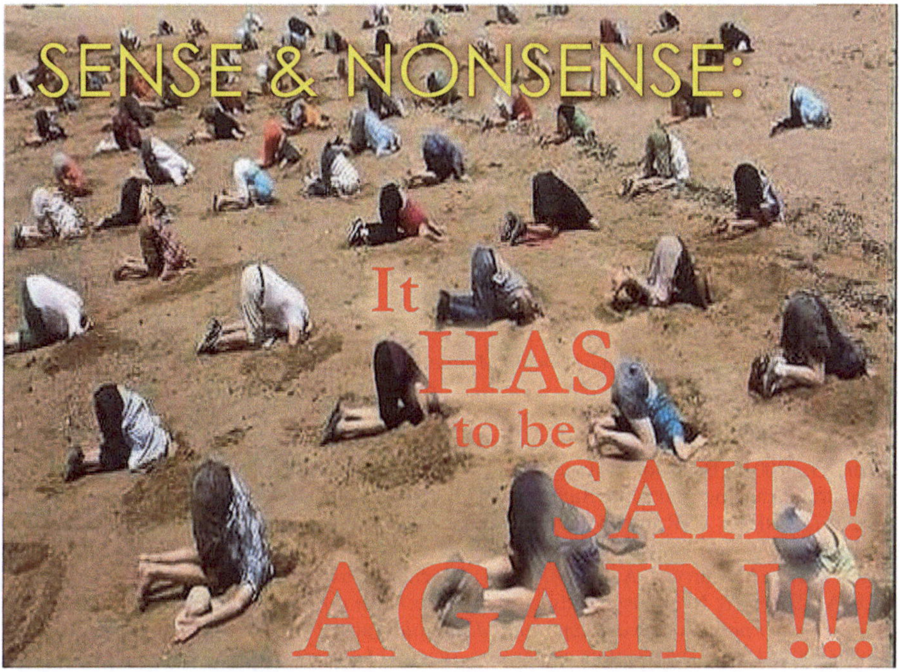

Fig. 2.37 It Has to Be Said–Again

as a selling point for ABA. But the reality is that a significant subset of children can achieve "recovery." Maybe we should use a different term than recovery, but if a child's IQ is in the normal range, if they are in general education, and they do not present with autism, call it what you want; but it is a very significant outcome!

There is no Lovaas model, plain and simple. Obedience and set protocols drive us crazy.

And, finally, and probably most importantly, not using qualified practitioners is INSANITY. We fully understand that there is a need for therapists. We get it, but we would not let a flight attendant fly a plane with the pilot checking in on her every now and then (Leaf et al., In Press). We would not have a school nurse do surgery. In the same way, we must have qualified interventionists doing intervention. We have had an office in England for 15 years. Initially, services were funded by the local educational authorities. After a few years, they stopped funding services. Why? Because they did a study in which unqualified therapists provided intervention and naturally the results demonstrated that "ABA was ineffective." So for years ABA was not funded until people began to understand the effectiveness of ABA is dependent upon the training of the interventionist.

Finally, our interpretation of the Lovaas model is that by providing the highest quality of therapy children with ASD can make amazing progress! I hope these before and after video clips will demonstrate the progress that children can make. You will see the first few minutes of intervention and then 10 weeks later:

VIDEO CLIP #8: http://www.autismpartnership.com/post/video-links-lovaas-model

And here are the same children 2 years later:

VIDEO CLIP #9: http://www.autismpartnership.com/post/video-links-lovaas-model

Thank you so much for coming and listening. I greatly appreciate it and I am so honored to be on a panel with these presenters. I know it is going to be a great day listening to them, as well. Thank you so much.

References

Baer, D. M. (2002). *Celebration of Donald M. Baer*. Paper presented at the celebration of Donald M. Baer, Lawrence, Kansas.

Chance, P., & Lovaas, I. (1974). After you hit a child, you can't just get up and leave him; You are hooked to that kid. Conversation with Ivar Lovaas. *Psychology Today, 7*, 76–84.

Green, G. (2001). Behavior analytic instruction for learners with autism advances in stimulus control technology. *Focus on Autism and Other Developmental Disabilities, 16*, 72–85.

Hart, B., & Risley, T. R. (1975). Incidental teaching of language in the preschool. *Journal of Applied Behavior Analysis, 8*, 411–420.

Hayes, L. J., & McCurry, C. A. (1990). Moral and scientific aspects of the punishment controversy. In A. C. Repp & N. N. Singh (Eds.), *Perspectives of the use of nonaversive and aversive interventions for persons with developmental disabilities* (pp. 87–102). Sycamore, IL: Sycamore.

Ito, R. (2004, April). The phantom chaser. *Los Angeles Magazine*, 50–57.

Kassardjian, A., Leaf, J. B., Ravid, D., Leaf, J. A., Alcalay, A., Dale, S., ... Oppenheim-Leaf, M. L. (2014). Comparing the teaching interaction procedure to social stories: A replication study. *Journal of Autism and Developmental Disorders, 44*, 2329–2340.

Leaf, J. B., Kassardjian, A., Oppenheim-Leaf, M. L., Cihon, J. H., Taubman, M., Leaf, R., & McEachin, J. (2016). Social thinking®: Science, pseudoscience, or antiscience? *Behavior Analysis in Practice.*

Leaf, J. B., Leaf, J. A., Alcalay, A., Dale, S., Kassardjian, A., Tsuji, K., ... McEachin, J. (2014) Comparison of most-to-least to error correction to teach tacting to two children diagnosed with autism. *Evidence-Based Communication Assessment and Intervention, 7*, 124–133.

Leaf, J. B., Leaf, R., Alcalay, A., Leaf, J. A., Ravid, D., Dale, S., ... Oppenheim-Leaf, M. (2015). Utility of formal preference assessments for individuals diagnosed with autism spectrum disorder. *Education and Training in Autism and Developmental Disabilities, 50*, 199–212.

Leaf, J. B., Leaf, R., McEachin, J., Taubman, M., Ala'i-Rosales, S., Ross, R. K., ... Weiss, M. J. (2016). Applied behavior analysis is a science and, therefore, progressive. *Journal of Autism and Developmental Disorders, 46*, 720–731.

Leaf, J. B., Leaf, R., McEachin, J., Taubman, M., Smith, T., Harris, S. L., ... & Waks, A. (In Press). Concerns about the registered behavior technician™ in relation to effective autism intervention. *Behavior Analysis in Practice.*

Leaf, J. B., Leaf, R., Taubman, M., McEachin, J., & Delmolino, L. (2014). Comparison of flexible prompt fading to error correction for children with autism spectrum disorder. *Journal of Developmental and Physical Disabilities, 26*, 203–224.

Leaf, R. B., & McEachin, J. J. (1999). *A work in progress: Behavior management strategies and a curriculum for intensive behavioral treatment of autism.* New York, NY: Different Roads to Learning.

Leaf, R. B., & McEachin, J. (2008). The UCLA Young Autism Project (YAP). In R. Leaf, J. McEachin, & M. Taubman (Eds.), *Sense and nonsense in the behavioral treatment of autism: It has to be said.* New York, NY: Different Roads to Learning.

Leaf, R. B., McEachin, J. J., & Taubman, M. (2008). *Sense and nonsense in the behavioral treatment of autism: It has to be said.* New York, NY: DRL Books.

Leaf, J. B., Oppenheim-Leaf, M. L., Call, N. A., Sheldon, J. B., Sherman, J. A., Taubman, M., … Leaf, R. (2012). Comparing the teaching interaction procedure to social stories for people with autism. *Journal of Applied Behavior Analysis, 45*, 281–298.

Leaf, J. B., Oppenheim-Leaf, M. L., Leaf, R. B., Taubman, M., McEachin, J., Parker, T., … Mountjoy, T. (2015). What is the proof? A methodological review of studies that have utilized social stories. *Education and Training in Autism and Developmental Disabilities, 50*, 127–141.

Leaf, J. B., Sheldon, J. B., & Sherman, J. A. (2010). Comparison of simultaneous prompting and no-no prompting in two-choice discrimination learning with children with autism. *Journal of Applied Behavior Analysis, 43*, 215–228.

Leaf, R. B., Taubman, M. T., McEachin, J. J., Leaf, J. B., & Tsuji, K. H. (2011). A programmatic description of a community-based intensive behavioral intervention program for individuals with autism spectrum disorders. *Education and Treatment of Children, 34*, 259–285.

Leaf, J. B., Tsuji, K. H., Griggs, B., Edwards, A., Taubman, M., McEachin, J., … Oppenheim-Leaf, M. L. (2012). Teaching social skills to children with autism using the cool versus not cool procedure. *Education and Training in Autism and Developmental Disabilities, 47*, 165–175.

Leaf, J. B., Tsuji, K. H., Lentell, A. E., Dale, S. E., Kassardjian, A., Taubman, M., … Oppenheim-Leaf, M. L. (2013). A comparison of discrete trial teaching implemented in a one-to-one instructional format and in a group instructional format. *Behavioral Interventions, 28*, 82–106.

Lipsker, L. E., Leaf, R. B., & Desio, C. L. (1978). *Good looking: A handbook of behavior modification*. Los Angeles, CA: Unpublished Manual.

Lovaas, O. I. (1981). *Teaching developmentally disabled children: The me book.* Austin, TX: PRO-ED Books.

Lovaas, O. I. (1987). Behavioral treatment and normal educational and intellectual functioning in young autistic children. *Journal of Consulting and Clinical Psychology, 55*, 3–9.

Lovaas, O. I., Koegel, R., Simmons, J. Q., & Long, J. S. (1973). Some generalization and follow-up measures on autistic children in behavior therapy. *Journal of Applied Behavior Analysis, 6*, 131–166.

Lovaas, O. I., Schaeffer, B., & Simmons, J. Q. (1965). Building social behavior in autistic children by use of electric shock. *Journal of Experimental Research in Personality, 1*, 99–109.

Lovaas, I. O., & Simmons, J. Q. (1969). Manipulation of self-destruction in three retarded children. *Journal of Applied Behavior Analysis, 2*, 143–157.

Maurer, A. (1983). The shock rod controversy. *Journal of Clinical Child Psychology, 12*, 272–278.

McEachin, J. J., Smith, T., & Lovaas, O. I. (1993). Long-term outcome for children with autism who received early intensive behavioral treatment. *American Journal on Mental Retardation, 97*, 359–372.

Moser, D., & Grant, A. (1965, May). Screams, slaps and love. *Life, 58*(18), 90–101.

Phillips, E. L., Phillips, E. A., Fixsen, D. L., & Wolf, M. M. (1974). *The teaching-family handbook.* Lawrence, KS: University of Kansas Printing Service.

Schopler, E., Short, A., & Mesibov, G. (1989). Relation of behavioral treatment to "normal functioning": Comments on Lovaas. *Journal of Consulting and Clinical Psychology, 57*, 162–164.

Soluaga, D., Leaf, J. B., Taubman, M., McEachin, J., & Leaf, R. B. (2008). A comparison of flexible prompt fading and constant time delay for five children with autism. *Research in Autism Spectrum Disorders, 2*, 753–765.

Stokes, T. F., & Baer, D. M. (1977). An implicit technology of generalization. *Journal of Applied Behavior Analysis, 10*, 349–367.

Taubman, M. T., Leaf, R. B., McEachin, J. J., Papovich, S., & Leaf, J. B. (2013). A comparison of data collection techniques used with discrete trial teaching. *Research in Autism Spectrum Disorders, 7*, 1026–1034.

Townley-Cochran, D., Leaf, J. B., Taubman, M., Leaf, R., & McEachin, J. (2015). Observational learning of students diagnosed with autism: A review paper. *Review Journal of Autism and Developmental Disorders, 2*, 262–272.

Chapter 3
Early Start Denver Model

Sally Rogers

Some aspects of the Early Start Denver Model go back to 1981, when I began working in Denver at the University of Colorado Medical Center to create a preschool for children with autism using a developmental model. That original work was known as the Denver Model. From that time until now, I've worked with teams in Colorado, University of Washington, and the MIND Institute at UC Davis to build and improve interventions for young children with ASD. The Early Start Denver Model (ESDM) was created by a partnership between Dr. Geraldine Dawson and me, in a STAART center grant that she received from NIH. I'm very grateful to Geri, and also to Laurie Vismara, who worked with me during her postdoctoral training and beyond to elaborate a way of coaching parents in ESDM. And I'm very grateful to the funders, particularly NIMH, NIDCD, and NICHD, and to the US Department of Education, who gave us our big grants, and the many foundations, especially Autism Speaks, that have supported our smaller studies.

Overview of ESDM

Today I will be covering the bare bones of how you provide ESDM and the conceptual basis for it. Let's start with an overview of the most important characteristics of the Early Start Denver Model (ESDM) (Rogers & Dawson, 2010): *A Developmental Framework*. First of all, it has a developmental framework. The main principles and characteristics of the content of the instruction for children come from a developmental framework, and the characteristics of the adult–child relationship and the way that

S. Rogers, Ph.D. (✉)
UC Davis, Mind Institute, Davis, CA, USA
e-mail: sjrogers@ucdavis.edu

R.G. Romanczyk, J. McEachin (eds.), *Comprehensive Models of Autism Spectrum Disorder Treatment*, DOI 10.1007/978-3-319-40904-7_3

we approach language comes from the science of developmental psychology. We understand autism as a developmental disorder, a brain-based disorder that affects virtually all areas of early childhood development.

The curriculum follows developmental sequences in multiple developmental domains in early childhood, covering developmental milestones that are acquired beginning at about age 9 months to about age 48 months, and we work within those development domains to choose developmental targets for learning. There is a concept from Vygotsky, which talks about the "zone of proximal development" (Vygotsky, 1978). It is a concept in developmental psychology that involves children's readiness to quickly learn certain skills, more than others, based on their current skill level and what lies just ahead in terms of typical developmental sequences. One study that demonstrated very nicely the importance of teaching skills in developmental sequence was carried out by Karen Lifter in the 90s (Lifter, Sulzer-Azaroff, Anderson, & Cowdery, 1993). She showed, in a single subject design, that teaching symbolic play using applied behavior analysis techniques resulted in rapid acquisition when steps were taught following typical developmental sequences, and when taught out of developmental sequence, resulted in very poor progress. This indicates the importance of evaluating children's areas of current skill development in terms of developmental sequences in order to identify the next skills that they are most "ready", or prepared, in terms of current abilities, to learn.

And, finally, the developmental concept looks at infant/toddler learning in terms of a number of characteristics that are quite different from learning that we see in older children and children who are both verbal and older. We see that infant/toddler learning is very affected by the quality of relationship with the adult and the sensitivity and responsivity of the adult to child cues and communications. It is also quite affected, particularly language learning, by adult characteristics which involve following the child's focus of attention, rather than redirecting and refocusing child attention (Tomasello, 1992). Thus, both of these characteristics—quality of relationships and following child attention rather than only directing it—are very important in our intervention, which is focused on very early childhood development.

Exploratory Nature of Infants. Another aspect of infant/toddlers that we value and want to support is the exploratory, active, hands-on nature of infant learning. Evolutionarily, we assume that for the young of our species and many others, this is a characteristic that allows them to have as many learning opportunities as possible at a time in which their brain and skill repertoires are maximally plastic and maximally being shaped by environmental experiences (Bower, 1989).

We see child initiative and exploration as a very important contribution of the child to his or her own learning, and we do everything we can to support and promote child initiative and spontaneity because we feel like we will never be able to deliver all the learning opportunities they need to catch up to their peers. We need their energy and action so that they can become self-generating learners and eventually can begin constructing their own learning experiences from their interactions in their social environment. Young children are multi-modal learners and the multiple sensory experiences that they have as they handle things, act on things, move things around, look, and listen provide many more learning opportunities than we adults can invent, and so we try to incorporate the child's own interests and preferences into the learning activities that we provide (Tanaka, Fukushima, Okanoya, & Myowa-Yamakoshi, 2014).

However, we also understand autism as a disorder in which specific areas of early childhood learning are most affected by the biology of autism and those include, unfortunately, all of the characteristics that allow children to learn easily from other people. **Social interest, preference for looking at social stimuli over others, social initiative**—these are decreased in early autism compared to any other group of children with developmental disorders (Dawson et al., 2004). **Imitation** skills are both immature and of very low frequency in early autism, compared to any other kind of learner (Rogers, Hepburn, Stackhouse, & Wehner, 2003). **Joint attention** behavior occurs out of sequence, it is very delayed and, it is very erratic in its appearance (Carpenter, Pennington, & Rogers, 2002). Many young children with ASD show very little joint attention, which is a critical skill, which we will come back to when we discuss communication development. **Both nonverbal and verbal communications** are significantly delayed, both expressively and receptively. Both **play skills with objects and pretend play** are negatively affected by autism (Sigman & Ungerer, 1984). These are the tools that young children use to learn from other people, and if a young child with autism cannot develop these social learning tools, they are not going to be able to learn easily from the social environment and they may end up on a very different course of learning, one that focuses on the objects in the environment rather than the people, throughout their lives. We feel very pressed by the knowledge of infant brain plasticity and the importance of shaping an infant brain into a social learning brain. These social learning tools are the building blocks that the child needs in order to become a skilled social learner.

An Integrated Whole. Another characteristic about the Early Start Denver Model is that it fuses three different areas of science and practice into an integrated whole in the treatment, and those three areas are developmental science including communication development, relationship-based science, and the learning science which applied behavior analysis represents. We don't see that developmental and behavioral approaches have to be in conflict; we see that these can be coordinated in terms of content and practice and we feel that we have fused them in our conceptualization of the treatment, in our approach to individualized intervention plans for each child, and in our ongoing interactions with children.

A Transdisciplinary Team. Another characteristic is that we work from a transdisciplinary team but using a generalist model. We see autism as affecting all areas of development, and we feel like we need the expertise of people who are skilled in motor development, communication development, skilled in education, skilled in relationships, skilled in applied behavior analysis—all areas affected by autism. These professionals are on the team and take a consultant role supporting the child's team leader, the team member who is taking the generalist model for a specific child, responsible for developing the treatment plan, assuring it is carried out, revising it as necessary, and partnering with the family to organize, direct, and supervise all the treatment that goes on.

In ESDM there is a primary therapist, who may be from any discipline. That person is a professional in their field. They are licensed with credentials according to their discipline, with a terminal degree. They have plenty of years of experience in early childhood and years of experience in autism. They are certified as an ESDM therapist and a parent coach and they manage all aspects of the work with the child. When they need expertise and consultation, they turn to the other people on the team, all of whom have evaluated the child, all of whom have followed the progress data, all of whom are involved in setting treatment plans and are continually aware of child progress and needs. This team meets weekly to review child progress. This is how we operate: the parent and the team leader are in the center together, planning and overseeing everything that is being carried out. If paraprofessionals are involved, they are supervised by that team leader, and the other disciplinary experts on the team are providing consultation for that team leader, while each of them is also a generalist team leader for other children. In this way, each team leader carries out an intervention that's transdisciplinary and the parent has only one person who is guiding them, which we think is absolutely critical to maximize child progress.

Multiple Methods of Delivery. Another characteristic of ESDM is that there is no one delivery system that is required. We have studied more intensive interventions, using one-on-one treatment at home plus parent coaching. We have supported children in preschool or daycare with one of our therapists accompanying them to help them learn in their natural settings. We have studied short-term parent delivery models in which weekly coaching is the only intervention. We also know various therapists who use ESDM as an individual therapy model: speech pathologists using ESDM as the frame within which they are treating children with autism, occupational therapists, physical therapists, psychologists, and behavior analysts. These all involve parent coaching because they are low-intensity interventions. And finally, we now have several published papers from group programs and day care centers, which go back to the origins of the Denver Model. We have seen group delivery involving inclusive settings and specialized settings, which include parent coaching as part of the model. The child's treatment plan is written to be embedded into natural routines using everyday materials and a naturalistic intervention style, which allows for this flexibility of delivery. It can be delivered any place where children are. We focus on routines and doing activities. I'll come back to that in a minute because that is really the vehicle within which young children are learning most of their skills. These are the basic elements of ESDM, descriptively.

Conceptual Basis of ESDM

One core idea is that intentional communication begins long before speech develops, that intentional communication begins in the child's sense of other people and themselves as a mind, as a person who generates goals and has plans and intentions and that you can anticipate someone's behavior in terms of their goals and that young children start learning to read other people's goals and intentions, their feelings, their communications in the 8–12-month period (Bretherton & Bates, 1979).

This is what the joint attention behaviors reflect—the preverbal toddler's understanding that another person has a mind and that one has to capture the partner's attention in order to get a message across, that two people can have a shared experience.

According to current communication science, this is a primary function of communication—to share experiences with another, and the child's earliest communicative gestures—pointing, giving, showing, sharing objects and emotions—those demonstrate the child's awareness of this. This is a conceptual core of our work in ESDM—that this is extremely challenging in early ASD and that we need to help the young children experience this in order to provide them with the interpersonal foundations for speech and language development. Thus, our activities with young children with ASD are built to emphasize this idea of self and other as a coordinated two-of-a-kind and that communication flows back and forth and that signals flow back and forth through simple body signals, that the child can begin to read, and through them, to begin to anticipate what people do and how they feel, think, and act.

A second core idea is that the quality of the child's individual relationship with their partner affects a child learning from that partner. Key characteristics of children's most successful relationships are with partners who are sensitive to the child's experiences and responsive to the child's cues (Thompson, 2000).

This requires that adults follow children's leads and are in a balanced, dyadic relationship with the child. If the child and the adult are partners in play, the adult is not primarily in a teacher role and the child is not primarily in a responsive role. The two of them are partners and they share directing and responding to each other. They take turns back and forth in the play. In the adult, turn is the opportunity to present a learning challenge to the child and in the child turn is the opportunity to establish a communication with the adult and assume that the adult is going to receive it. Child opportunities to lead represent child social initiations and spontaneous communications and intentional acts towards others—two characteristics that are often diminished in early autism.

A third core concept comes from the independent work of two developmental scientists, Peter Mundy, Ph.D., and Geraldine Dawson, Ph.D., who have suggested that autism reflects a biological impairment in the social attention and/or reward system, that people and social experiences are not as salient, or reinforcing for infants and young children with autism as they are for most children, and that because of this, they are less interested in interaction, receive back less reinforcement, and have fewer learning opportunities (Dawson, Meltzoff, Osterling, Rinaldi, & Brown, 1998; Mundy, 1995). This decrement in learning opportunities amasses hour-by-hour and day-by-day and results in growing developmental delays over time, which to some extent we believe reflect this lack of experience.

We want to prevent or lessen disability in children, development disability of any kind (Rogers & Dawson, 2010). Our three main goals are:

1. To bring children back into social interaction throughout their waking hours, as are all normally developing toddlers. If it takes 12 h a day for a little child without any difficulties to become a competent adult in our current society, then certainly a little child with autism is going to need the same 12 h a day in interaction to at

least be on the same playing field as the typically developing child. In ESDM, we are trying to level the playing field by getting massive amounts of learning opportunities delivered within social learning routines.
2. To teach children the building blocks of social learning: imitation, joint attention, play and pretend play, and language and nonverbal communication so that they can learn from others.
3. We need to fill in the learning gaps that they already have as fast as we can through intensive teaching, before they fall even farther behind.

Those are our main goals. Our interventions are also very strongly focused on social reinforcement and other reinforcements embedded in social activities with preferred materials. We want to increase learning rates, build repertoires of social communication and every other kind of skill, and prevent the experiential alterations that can so affect infant learning and, I assume, brain development and later capacity to process, deeply, language, social interaction, empathy, and the areas in which many adults with autism still struggle. That is the conceptual base of ESDM.

Primary Procedural Components of ESDM

Now we are moving to the procedural pieces of the intervention. The treatment procedures are detailed in the ESDM Manual authored by Rogers and Dawson (2010). In a nutshell, we assess, we write a treatment plan, and we deliver the treatment plan. Every 12 weeks, we reassess. Starting from scratch, we write a new treatment plan, we deliver that treatment plan, and at 12 weeks, assess it. This is the quarterly cycle that we use to carry out the intervention. Now I will describe the pieces inside that plan.

Assess Needs and Strengths

The assessment procedure that we use for all children involves the ESDM Curriculum Checklist. The tool and its usage are described in our treatment manual (Rogers & Dawson, 2010) for therapists, in which all the items are described, the assessment approach is laid out, and the scoring procedures explained. The data from the assessment, combined with parents' goals (the assessment includes parents), and data from other assessors as applicable, becomes the basis for building the treatment plan. We assess each child every 12 weeks on this curriculum. Whether they are getting 1 h a week of therapy or 25 h a week of therapy, they all get new objectives every 12 weeks.

The assessment procedure is set up around a series of play activities. Our goal is to get a picture of the child's skills inside typical routines and interactions, which is how the assessment is organized. The therapy room is set up like a playroom. There is a bean bag on the floor, carpeting, a couch, coffee table, two side chairs, and a small dining table and four chairs. There is a little child's table with chairs that fit the child, and there are a few toys on the table, some toys on the floor, and a couple of toys on the coffee table, adjacent to the couch and the side chairs. All the materials I need for this assessment—typical toys and everyday materials—are in the room in toy cabinets and on shelves. The child comes in with parents, sees familiar materials around, and frequently approaches materials after they have entered the room and settled in for a minute. We follow child interest in activities or if they are not approaching materials, we simply offer things, seeing what they are interested in doing. They start to play. We start to take a look at what they are doing, what their motor skills are like, and what their communication skills are like. We are interacting, like an adult would play with a toddler. How do they respond to me? There is the data for the social part of the scale.

We play together in an activity and when that is done, we start another activity. In so doing, we work our way through books and music and rhythm band instruments, and art activities, and bubbles, and balls, and snack time, and probably take shoes and socks on and off at some point to look at dressing. We just keep creating activities and keep filling up the curriculum based on what we are seeing and what the parent is telling us until we have established a basal and ceiling. We want to know where the child's basal and ceiling abilities are on each of the domains, so we include gross motor, fine motor, social, receptive language, expressive language, joint attention play, symbolic play, object play, imitation, etc. We are looking at a point within each of these domains that the child has mastered. Then we work to figure out where the "p/f, p/f, p/f, or partial passes" are, and when there is a point at which nothing else is being passed—we are at the ceiling of their abilities. Now we see the points at which this child goes from solid to, "I'm not there yet," and there is our proximal zone of development that we want to try to move through in the next 12 weeks.

Our treatment plans are written to describe what skills we plan to teach the child in 12 weeks. This is very much a creative process—there is no specific protocol here in terms of what you write. We do not write objectives item by item. Instead, we look ahead in the curriculum to see what this child needs to learn and is well-prepared to learn in the next 12 weeks. We aim as far as we think we can get in 12 weeks and our goal is to move the child as quickly as we can through each of these domains.

The assessment is an informal, reciprocal interaction in which the parent(s) and I are sitting together with the child, chatting, playing, with the child, sharing information back and forth; I want this to be a low-key, very relaxed interaction. It's the first time that therapists meet families and it sets up what everything is going to be like, so this runs like a therapy session. It's relaxed, it's based on activities, and it follows children along. There is no pressure. Moms have plenty of chances to show us what their children can do and tell us what their children can do, and we take the data from them, as well as what we are seeing. Of course, we get to see lots of behavior in an hour or so of play (and feeding, changing, etc.) routines, so we have many opportunities to see children communicate, handle objects, move through space, and show us the skills they have.

Select and Sequence Goals

At the end of the curriculum assessment, we have the data we need to develop the child's treatment goals. The team leader—the head therapist—now develops the objectives that define where we want to be in 12 weeks, and we write from 12 to 25 objectives—2 to 4 per domain area—for a 12-week period. For children who are not getting much therapy, say an hour a week, we would probably write two objectives in each domain. If the child is getting more like 20–25 h of therapy, we will write more objectives—four or so per domain—because the child is going to run through them and the therapist needs more to do. We will write three or four objectives in a domain, particularly in areas that are a challenge for a child. The number of objectives varies, but we are addressing all the domains with at least a couple of objectives and we are aiming for what we think can be realistically accomplished in 12 weeks, given the child in front of us and the amount of therapy that is going to be received.

Format of objectives. When we write an objective, it generally defines a skill that will be both mastered and generalized across persons, settings, and materials in a 12-week period. We write objectives in a particular formula: context, antecedent, behavior, and criterion.

Context. Objectives often, but not always, begin a context statement, "When using something, when eating meals, when entering school, when playing sensory social games". This is optional, but it helps to know in what situations data should be taken and skills should be taught, for those skills which are situation-specific.

Antecedent phrase. It is surprising to me how seldom I see these in most written objectives from school and other therapists. It is critical to an objective in that it defines the discriminative stimulus that will eventually activate the target behavior. Intentional behaviors occur in response to some stimulus, and in order to teach a child a new skill, it has to be taught in response to the antecedent that will eventually activate the behavior. "When x occurs, child will do y" lays out the causal relation between the antecedent and the behavior, and we write objectives in that way to help the therapist(s), teachers, parents, and any other intervenor remember how to set up the learning opportunity. What about behaviors that do not have a specific environmental antecedent—spontaneous behaviors like spontaneous requests, greetings, initiation of play? These often have setting or context variables that are important. "When the child is hungry, when the child enters the free play area of preschool," but there is no antecedent, and the fact that the behavior is expected to occur spontaneously, without an environmental Sd, is written into the objective. Example: When the child is hungry, he will approach an adult and say, "I'm hungry," spontaneously, with eye contact, several times per week, at home and at preschool.

Behavioral clause. This states the target child behavior that will follow the antecedent. We state behaviors at a level of mastery to be, the skill is consistently and fluently performed and performed independently. If it seems unreasonable to expect that the child will perform the selected skill at this level in 12 weeks, then the skill selected is too difficult and a less difficult skill needs to be selected. Teaching to mastery is a very important part of ESDM, and a very motivating part for staff and family. Generalization is also a part of the behavioral statement, and we expect that the skill will be consistently and independently performed across varying materials, people, and settings.

Criterion. The criterion defines mastery, what level and consistency of performance needs to be observed to consider the objective as mastered. The measurement aspect of the criterion needs to fit the type of behavior being observed, the expectable level of performance for children this age, and to be easy to measure during a treatment session. We very often write criteria in terms of the proportion of successful responses children demonstrate given the number of opportunities they had to show the skill. It is easier to define mastery when the criterion is "4/5 opportunities" than it is when the criterion is "3 times per hour", because three times per hour does not reflect how many times the antecedent was presented. Three times per hour given ten opportunities in the hour is a low rate of responding. Four out of five opportunities demonstrate a much more consistent rate of responding, information which cannot be gained when only counting frequency of a behavior.

Here is an example of an objective in the social domain.

During sensory social routines, when the adult briefly pauses in any one of five routines, child will spontaneously communicate to continue the routine using vocalizations or gestures plus gaze, in three of four opportunities, with two or more partners, in two or more settings, for three consecutive days.

- Setting: During sensory social routines or games without objects,
- Antecedent: When the adult briefly pauses in the game,
- Behavior: Child will spontaneously communicate to continue the routine using vocalizations or gestures plus gaze,
- Mastery and generalization criteria: In three of four pauses, in five different routines, for three consecutive days, with two or more partners, in two or more settings.

So that is the basic framework for the objective. A child has 12–25 of these, addressing all the developmental domains.

Teaching steps. The child's objectives form the treatment plan for 12 weeks, but they do not communicate to the therapist how to actually teach the skill. There is one more step we do. We break each objective down into a sequence of teaching steps. We create a sequence that begins with the first step representing the child's current mastery level, which will become a maintenance step. This is identified from the current highest pass the child has on the curriculum checklist. This is important for us because we are going to alternate acquisition and mastered skills, in order to maintain high levels of motivation for children and to keep the child's stress down in therapy. So the maintenance skill is step one. The last step—often step 6—describes the mastery/generalization skill level and represents the behavior as described in the objective. Then steps 2–5 represent a sequence in which the skill is gradually becoming more independent (prompt fading), more consistent (increased frequency, decreasing errors), more accurate (shaping), or progressively generalized. Each step becomes a teaching goal of its own, and the therapist focuses on teaching each step to mastery, which for us means three consecutive sessions with the step mastered, at which point the next step becomes the target of teaching. Thus, on day 1, the therapist will be focusing on teaching step 2 of all objectives and also eliciting and rewarding step 1 performance to maintain the current level and to alternate between maintenance and acquisition. Once step 2 has been performed consistently, step 3 becomes the acquisition step and step 2 the maintenance skill, and so forth. We expect to see children make significant progress in a step in a week. They may not master it in a week, but we want to see movement in the data on the current acquisition step, every week, and that becomes an important point that we will come back to.

From steps to a data sheet. The steps for each objective literally become the data sheet by word processing them into a single document. On the data sheet, we highlight the current acquisition step, so that it is clear to the therapist what the target is. We take data on acquisition and maintenance for all the objectives worked on in a session, and we expect to teach all objectives in a session. We take interval data every 15 min, going through the data sheet and coding every objective that has been attempted in that 15 min. The data are not trial data but rather performance summary data, indicating whether the child consistently demonstrated the behavior defined at the target step, or consistently failed it, or showed a mixed performance, using the symbols plus, minus, or plus/minus. At the end of the hour, we tally this and put this into a sheet that represents the performance for the day on each objective. This is how we summarize the data and make decisions about when to move forward to the next step. We also take daily data on child behavior on a Likert-based scale. We capture what the child's general behavior was like in the session: worse than average, average, better than average, or excellent behavior for learning. Here is an example of a brief data sheet.

Data Sheet

EXPRESSIVE

Vocalization w/ intent to request objects or activities 5+xs 80% opps

	1	2	3	4	5	6	7
Raches for obj (b)							
Voc 1x							
Voc 2x							
Voc 3x							
Voc 4xs							
Voc 5+xs 80% opps across 3 diff adults, settings, and vocs 4 out of 5							

Ask for help by handing the objest to the adult 5+x per session

	1	2	3	4	5	6	7
1x fpp (b)							
1x ppp							
1x spont							
2-4xs 50% opps							
2-4xs 80% opps							
5xs 50% opps							
5+xs 80% opps across 3+ adults, settings, and help opps 4 out of 5 tx							

RECEPTIVE LANGUAGE

Points or pats to 3+ pics when adult asks "Where is ___?" or "Show me ___", 80% of opps

	1	2	3	4	5	6	7
Points or pats 1x fpp (b)							
Points or pats 1x ppp							
Points or pats 1x indep 50%							
Points or pats 1x indep 80%							
Points or pats 2x indep 80%							
Points or pats 3+x indep 80% across 3+ adults, items & books 4 out of 5							

SOCIAL INTERACTION

Responds to greeting with E.C., gesture &/or vocalization @ 1st opp

	1	2	3	4	5	6	7
E.C. (b)							
E.C. + wave fpp							
E.C. + wave ppp							
E.C. + wave spont							
E.C. + voc w/ vp							
E.C. + voc spont							

COGNITIVE

Matches 5+ pairs of identical pictures with 80% accuracy

	1	2	3	4	5	6	7
1-2 pairs fpp (b)							
1-2 pairs 50% opps							
1-2 pairs 80% opps							
3-4 pairs 50% opps							
3-4 pairs 80% opps							
5+pairs 80% opps 3+ adults, settings, and activities 4 out of 5 tx ssn							

PLAY SKILLS

Play appropriately with 8 or more different one-step toddler toys involving 5+ toys 80% opps

e.g shapes in shapesorter, balls in ball maze, pegs in peg bo	1	2	3	4	5	6	7
1 toy ppp (b)							
1 toy 50% opps							
1 toy 80% opp							
2-4 toys 80 % opps							
5-7 toys 80% opps							
8+ toys 80% opps across 3+ adults, toys, and settings 4 out of 5 tx ssn							

	15 min	30 min	45 min	60 min	1 hr 15 min	1 hr 30 min	1hr 45 min	AVG
BX								
Routine								

Behavior codes

1. Severe behavior (e.g. aggression, SIB, frequent/intense tamtrums
2. Mild Behavior (e.g. noncompliance, some tantrums but able to participate in activity
3. Some behavior problems (e.g. fussy, whiny, some noncompliance but able to participate in most of activity
4. No problem behavior but difficulty staying on tast
5. Compliant , on-task, working at ability level
6. Above average performance for child, pleasant, excited about activity

Routine Codes

G	Greeting	S	Snack
F	Floor Activity	Q	Quiet
R	Sensory Social Routine	T	Table Activity
O	Outside	C	Closing

Managing Behavior Problems

You've noticed so far I've only been talking about developing skills; I haven't talked about managing problem behavior yet. You are probably getting the idea that we are using naturalistic teaching approaches, like those seen in incidental teaching, in which children have a great deal of control, not full control; it's shared control (Koegel, Koegel, Harrower, & Carter, 1999; McGee & Daly, 2007). You know from the literature that use of incidental teaching procedures results in fewer problem behaviors than adult-directed teaching. Children have a lot of access to their reinforcers, are carrying out preferred activities, and have some control. We have learned that, very often, problem behaviors in therapy will reduce quickly in the first few weeks of using a naturalistic behavioral approach and so, as part of the initial assessment, we identify the problem behaviors, we take data on them, and we make an initial decision based on the question, "Is there significant risk of injury or damage associated with the problem behavior?" If the answer is no, we do not develop specific plans for changing that behavior at the very start of treatment. Instead, we keep frequency data on it while moving immediately into using ESDM as a naturalistic developmental-behavioral teaching approach (NDBI). If our data demonstrate that the identified problem behavior is decreasing, we continue with ESDM, coach parents, and others to use it and continue to keep data on the behavior until it is no longer a problem.

However, if the behavior problem is not decreasing in the first 2 or 3 weeks or if it is so difficult that we cannot engage the child, then we do a functional assessment and write a positive behavior support plan (PBSP) (Carr et al., 2002). This becomes part of the child's treatment plan, along with the child's objectives and steps, and it is implemented across all environments. Thus, the developmental learning plan and the behavior plan together form the child's curriculum.

This is the same process that we use if the answer to the, "Is there significant risk of injury or damage associated with the problem behavior?" question is yes. If the child does have dangerous behaviors, we immediately complete a functional assessment, develop a positive behavior support plan, and implement both the developmental plan and the positive behavior support plan and keep track of the frequency data for the problem behavior(s). If the frequency/severity is decreasing, we continue with our treatment as planned. If it is not decreasing, we immediately seek consultation among our team or outside our team to improve the PBSP. We expect to see behavior changes rapidly in problem behaviors and we take it very seriously if there is not a positive response. We have a behavior analyst on every team, and everybody on the team is well-trained in behavioral concepts as well.

Teach Inside Joint Activity Routines

Let's now talk about how we are going to implement teaching on the child's developmental learning objectives inside the therapy sessions. In ESDM, the frame for teaching is an activity. It's not an exchange and it is not a particular behavior. It is a whole activity: an art activity, a music activity, a book activity, a chase game, a dance activity, a puzzle activity, pretend play, bubbles, building with blocks or Legos, playing in water in the kitchen sink. An activity is also a routine: bedtime routines, chores, store routines, special events like a birthday party or Christmas, dressing routines, meal routines, toileting routines—these routines that mark children's lives. Activities of all types are the frames for ESDM teaching.

We create the activities for teaching by having families identify for us what the child's routines are at home, or what they wish were the child's routines at home, if the child would comply. Additionally, in our therapy hours, we build routines out of typical early childhood activities that this child would do in any daycare center, any toddler group, or any preschool. We use materials that exist in these settings; we do not construct materials. We use materials the child would run into in any pediatric office, any preschool, and at home, so that they know what to do with the materials they will encounter in everyday environments.

In creating everyday activities within which we will teach, we were greatly influenced by the work of Jerome Bruner and we evolved a structure from his work, which is spelled out in our manuals, treatment protocols, fidelity tools, etc. (Bruner, 1981). We are creating "Joint Activity Routines," and we define a joint activity routine first of all by its structure and second by its interactional style. Structurally, it has four steps:

There is a **setup** which begins at the first move made towards a new activity and continues until a theme emerges. The **theme** becomes the verb that you are doing. You might be making straight lines, you might be throwing, you might be twirling, you might be pointing at holes in a pegboard. Your theme is the action the child is doing, and the theme is marked by both repeated actions of the adult and the child accompanied by the language that the adult is using and the repetition of this behavior back and forth between the partners.

After a while, changes enter the theme, **variations in the theme** that need to come about as a child masters the theme. The variations are really important for a number of reasons: (a) It requires children to play with things in more than one way; it's building flexibility into play activities and social interactions from the beginning; it's building the child's repertoire of ways to handle this material from the beginning. (b) It also holds the child's attention by introducing novelty, which captures attention and keeps the play activity going longer. (c) It reduces repetitive actions.

Varying the theme of play activities and introducing multiple variations support one of the rules of ESDM: teaching multiple objectives inside every activity, multiple objectives from multiple domains. An additional rule is that in every activity, you are teaching social and/or communication objectives. In any one activity—art, books, puzzles, gross motor—you are teaching one or more objectives that are easily addressed in this activity, and in addition to that, you are also teaching social-communication objectives: gestures, communication, imitation, joint attention, language. Variations serve different developmental objectives and domains or learning and functions for the child with ASD as it does for typical toddlers, to address many different types of learning opportunity within an everyday activity. So the variations are important for flexibility, vocabulary, getting more objectives in, increasing play complexity, and increasing attention span.

The fourth and final step involves a **closing and transition**. The activity needs to finish. We want an orderly finish where the adult and child together are closing this play down and transitioning to some other activity. A well-done transition results in no stopping of learning opportunities from one activity to the next. In a well-done closing, you never lose the child's attention, you never stop interacting, and you move smoothly from one piece of play into another, maintaining your learning number of trials. A good therapist in ESDM averages a learning trial about every 10 s, and in order to keep the opportunities flowing, we need a smooth and interactive closing and new opening.

In each activity, you will carry out multiple objectives, and actually in each of the four parts of the activity you may have different objectives being taught, because different parts of the four-part joint activity routine may best support some objectives over others.

Addressing all objectives inside a therapy session. Another ESDM practice is that the therapist teaches all objectives inside a session. That means that between 12 and 24 skills are being practiced, multiple times, in an hour, which is intensive teaching. The use of the 4-step joint activity structure really helps therapists achieve this goal, because each step of the 4-step joint activity structure allows for teaching of several objectives, and the strategic use of various activities supports objectives in various domains. The ESDM practice of addressing multiple objectives in each activity is what allows for so much teaching of objectives to occur. Eight or nine activities in an hour, each with four parts, each part with multiple objectives, involve ample opportunities to work in all domains of early childhood development. Furthermore, the requirement that language/social communication objects are taught inside every activity assures a great deal of communication teaching to occur. Teaching multiple objectives inside each activity makes each activity last longer than it would have if only one skill, and one theme, were the focus, and this also helps intensify teaching. Longer activities, with fewer transitions, assure longer spans of child attention, which we need in order to teach. Longer activities are less exhausting for the adult and for the children, promoting longer periods of social attention and social engagement.

Interactive aspects of joint activity routines. We have been discussing the structure of a joint activity, but through this discussion, you probably also get a sense about the interactive quality of these routines. They involve play partners, with the child and the adult both engaged in the activity, co-constructing the activity. Each is adding ideas—themes—to the play, the child in his or her first action, the adult skilled in taking whatever the child does and playing back and forth together on the theme, imitating the theme, sharing the theme, taking turns on the theme, and then working variations in, which might come from the child and might come from the adult, and represent more opportunities for learning. The adult is playing back and forth, only occasionally directing, and following at least as often as leading. Having the child involved in choosing the materials and theme assures some positive value for the child, and having adults follow, imitate, and not direct adds further positive value. When the adult leads, the child's ability to regain control of the material maintains the reinforcing quality of the activity for the child. The reinforcer is in the child's ability to achieve his or her goals and that needs to be paired with the presence of the responsive social partner, who is imitating them and making it more fun—this is the social reward piece of the activity.

Tailoring the Teaching Approach to Individual Child Needs

I have been describing how we begin in ESDM, the way that we build the teaching plan and the style of teaching that we first use with each child. We take interval data on child performance every 15 min, and we expect to see progress in the data every week on the steps that are being taught. If we do not see progress, we assume there is a problem with our teaching plan and we start to adapt it. In order to do this, we apply the decision tree that is described in the Rogers & Dawson, 2010 ESDM manual. Why do we move to adapt the teaching plan so quickly? Because we do not want children, therapists, or parents to experience failure repeatedly and to become discouraged. We don't want children to develop an aversion to materials because they are not successful with them. If the child is not progressing rapidly, we focus on changing the variables, one at a time, to understand what adaptations to the teaching procedure will be most helpful for this individual child.

First, we focus on reinforcer strength. We may need to add other kinds of reinforcers that will deliver stronger rewards for targeted child behavior and, if we don't have an activity that has inherent reward value for an individual child (e.g., toilet training), we have to use other kinds of reinforcement anyway. So first, we focus on reinforcer strength. If strengthening reinforcers doesn't change the child's rate of learning, we start to add structure and repetition to the teaching situation. There are about six steps in the adaptation hierarchy, but basically we add more repetitions, take away variations in materials and, if we need to, we take away variations in physical set up for the teaching. The hierarchy moves all the way to discrete trial teaching and, if discrete trial teaching is the most helpful strategy for a child to learn a particular skill, this is how we will teach it. Whatever characteristics of teaching a child needs in order to make the most rapid progress, we make that adjustment and continue to teach that way for that objective until it's mastered, but only for that objective. We change teaching approaches for the objectives the child is struggling to learn and maintain those adaptations for 12 weeks, at which point we begin teaching a new set of objectives and again typically begin with naturalistic teaching.

Repeat Process Every 12 Weeks

Some children need the entire program delivered in a more structured way. If that is the case, we do it, but every 12 weeks we do the assessment in this more incidental way because, at some point, most children are going to have the skills and the interest to learn well from a naturalistic teaching approach, and we feel like we can get more teaching in—that we can just do a better job teaching—if we can use a naturalistic teaching approach. We would like to use it if it supports the child's most rapid learning, but we want to use whatever teaching approaches are most effective for an individual child's learning. The final alteration we make are visual supports, and it surprises many of our colleagues that we move to visual approaches as the last of our adaptations, but we do this because we feel that reward strength and effective teaching strategies are the primary ingredients for effective teaching, assuming that the teaching target is well-chosen, and therefore those are the first teaching elements that we individualize.

The Evidence Base

There are currently around 15 papers published on the Early Start Denver Model. The first study was a randomized controlled trial that Geraldine Dawson at the University of Washington conducted (Dawson et al., 2010) with 48 children who were 2-year-olds at the start of treatment. It was for this study that Geri and I worked together to create the ESDM. In the study, the team planned to deliver 24 months of 20 h-per-week of ESDM in children's homes, one-on-one, with paraprofessionals who were carefully supervised and trained by their professional team leader, who also provided biweekly parent coaching throughout the study. In that study, the ESDM group demonstrated quite significant gains in IQ, compared to children who had been randomized to a group receiving their treatments in the community. Unexpectedly, the community group averaged almost as many hours of intervention as the ESDM group received, so group differences were not due to treatment intensity. The study demonstrated an increase of over one standard deviation in IQ in the ESDM group. We found an 18-point increase in IQ in 2 years of treatment and a significant, more than one standard deviation, increase in language, both expressive language and receptive language gain, in the children who received ESDM compared to the community treatment group, and about a 3/4 of a standard deviation difference in Vineland overall scores in ESDM group compared to the community group. In multiple developmental domains, we saw a significant and large effect of ESDM.

We also found two areas of significant change in their ASD symptoms. First of all, we saw changes in their clinical diagnosis as rated by a study team of clinical psychologists blind to treatment group. For the majority of children in the ESDM group who changed diagnoses in terms of the DSM-IV diagnostic system, they changed from Autistic Disorder to PDD-NOS, which refers to milder symptoms. In the community group, the diagnoses that did change moved in the opposite direction, from PDD to Autistic Disorder, and the differences in these proportions were statistically significant.

We also gathered the PDD-BI index from teachers when the children were four and ending therapy and we found significant differences. The ESDM group showed more social approach behavior to peers than did the community treatment group, and the ESDM group showed less social avoidance and problems with peers than did the community treatment group.

Dawson et al. 2012, Geraldine Dawson and colleagues published a study looking at brain responses from these children to social and nonsocial stimuli. This paper represented the first study of brain effects of a behavioral intervention that had been published in autism research, so this was a very important study for all of us. Of course, we assume that when we are changing behavior we are changing brain function because brain function underlies all behavior, but no one had demonstrated it. Dawson demonstrated that after 2 years of treatment, the children who received ESDM showed much stronger electrical impulses, stronger and faster, to computerized pictures of female faces than they did to toys, and their response was indistinguishable from typically developing 4 year olds. The group who had received community treatment showed the opposite pattern: much stronger and faster electrical brain responses to toys than to faces, a pattern that had been previously associated with autism and discriminating of autism from other groups.

This is a big finding that demonstrates exactly what we are trying to do, all of us, to help shape young children's behavior and underlying bran responses into patterns in which social input, social partners, and social learning become the most important referents in their experiences. A Nobel Prize learning scientist and psychoanalyst, Eric Kandel (2007), stated in his fantastic book, *In Search of Memory*, that therapy works by altering the structure and function of the brain. He is talking about psychoanalysis, but in a broader sense he is talking about learning, and we are demonstrating it in this study of autism treatment. He says from his lifelong studies of animal learning that the mechanism underlying learning is the ability of neurons to change the strength and number of synapses in response to learning opportunities. That's what is happening in the trials that we are all doing. We are changing brain structure and function (chemistry) in the synapse between neurons. The more numerous those synaptic connections and neural networks are and the more wide-ranging they are, the more information children can process and the wider are the number of responses, words, ideas, and behaviors children bring to every moment that they are interacting with anyone as well as learning while playing alone. These are the neural products of our work with children with ASD.

We have demonstrated that the accelerated learning rate with these children in Washington is maintained 2 years after treatment ends. They gained another ten points in IQ and also continued to show significant advantages over the control groups in nonverbal learning rates, in rate of receptive vocabulary development, in their adaptive behavior skills, and in the severity of their autism symptoms.

This is without any further ESDM treatment after the 24 months had ended.

We also demonstrated that neither IQ nor language learning rate moderates the effect of ESDM. Children in lower and higher IQ groups both show similar proportion of rate gain. It's true for IQ; it's true for language.

However, the symptom severity of autism does affect the amount of gain that is made. Children with milder autism made more IQ gain in 2 years than children with more severe symptoms of autism. However, both groups significantly outperformed the community children in terms of their learning rates.

We also have the first controlled study of ESDM in groups, published by Vivanti and colleagues (2012) at La Trobe University in Melbourne, Australia. The children receiving ESDM in a group daycare center for a 12-month period made significant gains in IQ, language, and adaptive behavior compared to a well-matched comparison group of children attending a publicly funded autism specialty program in the same community.

Parents like ESDM delivery and rate it highly compared to other kinds of therapy they are getting. They tell us they feel like their working alliances with ESDM therapists are particularly strong. We have a cost analysis study, done by David Mandel, which demonstrates that the cost-benefit starts to re-accrue the cost of ESDM within 3 years from the start of the 24-month treatment. In the Dawson et al. (2010) study, Mandell found that the ESDM group was receiving fewer specialized services and that the sumtotal of funds expended for care was less for the ESDM group across those 3 years than it was for the community group even though the children who had received ESDM for 24 months were significantly out-performing their peers receiving community intervention.

Summary

In this chapter, we have reviewed the basic concepts and practices associated with the Early Start Denver Model, a naturalistic developmental-behavioral intervention. We have demonstrated that it is possible to fuse these two bodies of knowledge into an effective intervention that systematically addresses the content and the process of intervention and also allows for systematic individualization through the use of a decision tree that leads the therapist through a wide range of alternative empirically supported teaching practices in order to best address the child's learning style. We have discussed the flexible nature of the delivery of ESDM, its use in natural environments, everyday routines, and everyday materials. We have discussed building and delivering the treatment plan, use of motivational strategies, and management of problem behavior.

In closing, I want to refer to a quote from Alfred Adler, "The child is both the artist and the painting". This captures well the developmentalist concept that children construct their own learning opportunities, and in so doing, build their own individual personalities, strengths, interests, and talents, while at the same time they represent the products of their community of careers' and teachers' efforts. This demonstrates how we have constructed ESDM for early autism treatment, to help children develop the tools they need to construct their own learning opportunities and learn from others.

Disclosures I receive royalties for materials I have written and for materials I have created for training. I receive honoraria for talks that I give.

References

Bower, T. G. (1989). *The rational infant: Learning in infancy*. New York: WH Freeman/Times Books/Henry Holt.

Bretherton, I., & Bates, E. (1979). The emergence of intentional communication. *New Directions for Child and Adolescent Development, 1979*(4), 81–100.

Bruner, J. (1981). The social context of language acquisition. *Language & Communication, 1*(2), 155–178.

Carpenter, M., Pennington, B. F., & Rogers, S. J. (2002). Interrelations among social-cognitive skills in young children with autism. *Journal of Autism and Developmental Disorders, 32*(2), 91–106.

Carr, E. G., Dunlap, G., Horner, R. H., Koegel, R. L., Turnbull, A. P., Sailor, W., … Fox, L. (2002). Positive behavior support evolution of an applied science. *Journal of Positive Behavior Interventions, 4*(1), 4–16.

Dawson, G., Jones, E. J., Merkle, K., Venema, K., Lowy, R., Faja, S., … Smith, M. (2012). Early behavioral intervention is associated with normalized brain activity in young children with autism. *Journal of the American Academy of Child & Adolescent Psychiatry, 51*(11), 1150–1159.

Dawson, G., Meltzoff, A. N., Osterling, J., Rinaldi, J., & Brown, E. (1998). Children with autism fail to orient to naturally occurring social stimuli. *Journal of Autism and Developmental Disorders, 28*(6), 479–485.

Dawson, G., Rogers, S., Munson, J., Smith, M., Winter, J., Greenson, J., … Varley, J. (2010). Randomized, controlled trial of an intervention for toddlers with autism: the Early Start Denver Model. *Pediatrics, 125*(1), e17–e23.

Dawson, G., Toth, K., Abbott, R., Osterling, J., Munson, J., Estes, A., & Liaw, J. (2004). Early social attention impairments in autism: social orienting, joint attention, and attention to distress. *Developmental Psychology, 40*(2), 271–283.

Kandel, E. R. (2007). *In search of memory: The emergence of a new science of mind*. New York: WW Norton.

Koegel, L. K., Koegel, R. L., Harrower, J. K., & Carter, C. M. (1999). Pivotal response intervention I: Overview of approach. *Research and Practice for Persons with Severe Disabilities, 24*(3), 174–185.

Lifter, K., Sulzer-Azaroff, B., Anderson, S. R., & Cowdery, G. E. (1993). Teaching play activities to preschool children with disabilities the importance of developmental considerations. *Journal of Early Intervention, 17*(2), 139–159.

McGee, G. G., & Daly, T. (2007). Incidental teaching of age-appropriate social phrases to children with autism. *Research and Practice for Persons with Severe Disabilities, 32*(2), 112–123.

Mundy, P. (1995). Joint attention and social-emotional approach behavior in children with autism. *Development and Psychopathology, 7*, 63–82.

Rogers, S. J., & Dawson, G. (2010). *Early start Denver model for young children with autism: Promoting language, learning, and engagement*. New York: Guilford Press.

Rogers, S. J., Hepburn, S. L., Stackhouse, T., & Wehner, E. (2003). Imitation performance in toddlers with autism and those with other developmental disorders. *Journal of Child Psychology and Psychiatry, 44*(5), 763–781.

Sigman, M., & Ungerer, J. A. (1984). Cognitive and language skills in autistic, mentally retarded, and normal children. *Developmental Psychology, 20*(2), 293.

Tanaka, Y., Fukushima, H., Okanoya, K., & Myowa-Yamakoshi, M. (2014). Mothers' multimodal information processing is modulated by multimodal interactions with their infants. *Scientific Reports, 4*, 6623.

Thompson, R. A. (2000). The legacy of early attachments. *Child Development, 71*(1), 145–152.

Tomasello, M. (1992). The social bases of language acquisition. *Social Development, 1*(1), 67–87.

Vivanti, G., Dissanayake, C., Zierhut, C., Rogers, S. J., & Victorian ASELCC Team. (2012). Brief report: Predictors of outcomes in the Early Start Denver Model delivered in a group setting. *Journal of Autism and Developmental Disorders, 43*(7), 1717–1724.

Vygotsky, L. S. (1978). *Mind in society: The development of higher mental process*. Cambridge, MA: Harvard University Press.

Chapter 4 The New England Center for Children: Applied Behavior Analysis for Treating All Levels of ASD Severity

William H. Ahearn

Introduction

The New England Center for Children has provided services to individuals with autism and related disabilities for about 40 years. We are very different from the first two service providers that spoke at this conference and very different from Mark Sundberg's service delivery in that we are a private nonprofit school for individuals with autism and related disabilities. You will see, however, there are many similarities in terms of the approach. There are some differences, as well. As I go along, there were a number of specific aspects about service delivery that Ray was very insistent that we all hit upon, as mentioned in the introduction and the first two presenters were excellent in hitting upon those; I am going to as well. Some of what I would like to thread through, in terms of our differences, may at some point seem like I am disagreeing with something that someone else has said, but more of what I am attempting to do is lay things out a little differently in terms of what it is that we do at the New England Center for Children (NECC), and you will see if you follow along for a while where those commonalities come in and the structured approach. NECC was founded by Vincent Strully in Massachusetts at a time when the deinstitutionalization movement for persons with special needs was gaining traction. There was strong support from the state government, particularly from Governor Mike Dukakis, to foster appropriate services, especially for those with severe problem behavior. Vinnie had come into contact with behavior analysis and believed strongly that applied behavior analysis was the best route to developing effective treatment.

W.H. Ahearn, Ph.D., BCBA-D (✉)
The New England Center for Children, Southborough, MA, USA
e-mail: bahearn@necc.org

R.G. Romanczyk, J. McEachin (eds.), *Comprehensive Models of Autism Spectrum Disorder Treatment*, DOI 10.1007/978-3-319-40904-7_4

Overview of NECC

The scope of services provided by NECC is broad. Like the other service providers presenting at this conference, we also provide the early intensive behavioral intervention (EIBI) that has been widely recognized as the most effective means of treating autism (see Ahearn & Tiger, 2012). Home-based services are the primary setting in which we currently provide EIBI though historically we have also provided these in our central facility. Our home-based program has around 36 students receiving services. The center-based services that we provide are housed near Boston in Southborough, Massachusetts, and we have a replication site in Abu Dhabi (for more specific and up-to-date information on services, visit https://www.necc.org/). For these center-based services, there are different ways that people are accessing them. There is a segment of those who we are serving that live at home and come in to receive day services as if they were going to school in their home district. Currently, we have about 90 students in the Boston-based day services, whereas over in Abu Dhabi, we are serving about 120 individuals in those day services and that is our primary service delivery that is occurring in Abu Dhabi. The next tier of service provision is residential services, and the majority of the individuals coming into residential programming have severe problem behavior. Most of these individuals have not been able to be safely managed or have suffered significant worsening of their problem behavior in their home and school environments leading to the need for intensive services. The severity of problem behavior presenting in our day services students has significantly increased over the past decade or so as more behavior analytic services have become available in Massachusetts. This had led to many children with autism being able to remain in their home school districts and receive effective educational and clinical services.

I want to spend a little bit of time on the structural systems that we have dealing with severe problem behavior (treatment is function focused as described below) and how that is integrated into our services at NECC. The number of students in our residential services is about 130, 86 of which receive staff-intensive funding. The students that are in our residential program live in houses in the metro-west area of Boston and are transported by our staff to the central facility. There are typically 8–9 students in each residential unit with a team of teachers/therapists providing treatment in both the residential and school setting. As I mentioned these students have severe problem behavior but there is severe problem behavior, and then there is extremely severe problem behavior. Self-injury and aggression are common in persons with autism and are substantial challenges for clinicians; however, when not treated effectively early in life or as the child ages, we sometimes observe a level of severity in which the individual's well-being is significantly and frequently compromised. This is reflected in the resources necessary to safely and effectively treat problem behavior. Our most resource-intense services are our staff-intensive residential services. These students present with severe problem behavior best characterized as intractable problem behavior. Our staff-intensive unit resides in specially designed housing with four adjoining apartments where there are a total of 27 staff-intensive funded students. We also have public school classrooms, or what we refer to as our partner program, where we are currently running 27 classrooms with an average of about six students in each of those classrooms, so I think the total is somewhere around 180 students receiving services through us in public school. Obviously, if you can keep students in their home school districts, you are saving a substantial amount of money relative to sending them to a specialized facility, so obviously serving those individuals there meets the needs of the community and, hopefully, the needs of each of those individuals. NECC also provides consultative services to somewhere in the neighborhood of 600 students.

Conceptual Basis of NECC's Approach

In terms of the basis for our approach, it is, as mentioned above, behavior analysis. However, many misrepresent or do not accurately grasp behavior analysis. Applied behavior analysis (ABA) is the application of those principles of behavior analysis, while the conceptual foundation for both behavior analysis and applied behavior analysis is Skinner's radical behaviorism (Skinner, 1945, 1953, 1957). To say that behaviorism, per se, is the foundation of behavior analysis, I think, is not entirely accurate because the reason why Skinner included that "radical" in front of behaviorism is because, at the time when he was developing his conceptual approach, Watson (1913) introduced a very important notion and that is science is important and it is the best way to come to an understanding of phenomena in the world. So psychology, if it is going to do anything useful according to Watson, needs to be a science. So that was an excellent idea, but there were a lot of problems with Watson's extreme environmentalism and very quickly that fell out of favor, and Hull's (1935) neobehaviorism gained prominence over Watson's approach.

At the same time, Tolman's (1938) purposive behaviorisms, or as some in psychology at the time like to refer to it "neoneobehaviorism," were schools of thought within psychology that were developing. However, distinct from those approaches is Skinner's radical behaviorism. Radically different, but what do you mean by radically different? Skinner's approach is that behavior occurs and has a function. The function of behavior is much more important for us in terms of interpreting its cause than is what it looks like. Just as an example, all of you are familiar with self-injurious behavior and topographical descriptions of self-injurious behavior. Those are not very useful when it comes to developing effective interventions for them. A functional approach, however, is one that is much more useful because it places behavior within the environmental context in which we encounter behavior (see Iwata, Dorsey, Slifer, Bauman, & Richman, 1994a, Iwata, Pace, et al., 1994b; Pelios, Morren, Tesch, & Axelrod, 1999). So that idea that was radical is that behaviorists functionally relate behavior to environmental events.

Skinner (e.g., 1950) makes a distinction between his radical behaviorism and psychology as a whole which he characterizes as being methodologically behaviorism. Psychology, from this view, treats behavior as an index for things going on in other places. His functional approach studies behavior per se in its own right, or as I like to think of we are studying "the things unto themselves." So in a science of behavior is very important for us to understand that we are looking at individuals and not brains. So as a clinician, you are a teacher, you are a behavioral analyst, you are a BCBA, and you are a licensed clinical psychologist with behavior analytic training; what you have in front of you is a person. You don't have a brain that you can see. From this perspective it does not matter to whether you have a brain or a 57 Chevy engine in the place of a brain. A clinician needs to deal with you and your behavior, right here, right now, and what the clinician sees in the context in which that behavior has developed over time.

This natural science approach is one that assumes that behavior occurs within a selectionist perspective (Skinner, 1981). What Skinner posited (see also Ahearn & Tiger, 2012) is that there are three levels of causality with respect to behavior. Firstly, there is phylogeny or the genetic inheritance that the individual walks into the door with. Secondly, there is their life experience or ontogeny, so learning occurs, both operant and respondent, and as we encounter an individual's behavior, we assume the genetic underpinnings, whereas we operate with assumption that there are both operant and respondent learning that have produced the behavior we observe. Respondent learning is important in its own right, and it is embedded within any three-term operant contingency. That is, the discriminative stimulus naturally correlates in time—it is temporally associated with—the consequences. Thus, what comes with that three-term contingency is not only an operant but also a respondent. So, in addition to the point at which we mostly acutely focus at the ontogenic or the life history level, there are sociocultural practices, as they influence how that individual learns and what they learn, say, and so forth. We talk about language and Mark Sundberg's chapter in this volume spends a lot of time covering this topic. On sociocultural influences on behavior, for example, when we have a young child who begins to babble, it does not matter whether they are babbling in China or Africa or the United States; the babbling is similarly undifferentiated with the same sorts of sounds. Differential reinforcement on the part of the social environment, particularly the caregivers, is what shapes and establishes the phonemes that then emerge within that individual's repertoire. So is it something naturally unfolding within the brain? No, it is the social practices that differentially reinforce those sounds that become part of that individual's repertoire. When the repertoire is defective, if we come at that challenge with this functional perspective, it allows us to direct teaching communication by shaping and establishing verbal behavior by addressing the purposes it serves in our verbal community. I posit that this is superior or to a structural approach focusing on definitions, grammar, and syntax.

Primary Procedural Components

The next area each speaker was asked to discuss was what the primary procedural components of our approach are.

EIBI/ABA Through the Life Span

As mentioned previously, applied behavior analysis permeates all of NECC's services. For us it is not just early intensive behavioral intervention; rather, it is applied behavior analysis through the life span. So we typically have two things in front of us as applied behavior analysts when we encounter a person with autism, skill deficits, and behavioral excesses.

Skill Deficits

In terms of dealing with those skill deficits, we take a look at the function of those skills in the social environment from two perspectives: one, what is the function of that behavior for the typically developing child or the typically developing adult? Because that is what our target is, not to teach them to look at somebody. I could teach you to look at somebody's eyes. I have done this many times. I can get you from perseverative focus on lips to looking at eyes, but are you motivated to do that? That is the goal, to establish behavior under the appropriate motivative control. What is the circumstance that leads to that, when we see it in typically developing people relative to those that do not have that in their repertoire? So with that functional focus, that then leads us to specific targeting via appropriate teaching procedures in an attempt to establish those functions and not just the topographies of responses that need to be there. I'm going to give you some overt examples below.

Problem Behavior

In terms of problem behavior, there are four basic kinds of contingency classes (socially maintained positive reinforcement, socially maintained negative reinforcement, automatically maintained positive reinforcement, and automatically maintained negative reinforcement) that are found to maintain problem behavior. Integrating those contingencies with the motivational operations that overlay upon them, the context in which those problem behaviors occur, and the social environment that is supporting behavior, is very complex. For this reason functional behavioral assessment cannot typically be done in a very short period of time, and repeated observations are often necessary. So validated function-based treatment is something that is most likely the best way of dealing with problem behavior (Hanley, Iwata, & McCord, 2003). Therefore NECC's approach is heavily focused on teaching appropriate replacement behavior that matches the function of problem behavior.

How Goals Are Selected and Sequenced

Now, how are goals selected and sequenced at NECC? For a long time before we developed our Autism Curriculum Encyclopedia®, discussed in more detail below, we had a list of hierarchically ordered skills across several skill domains that we thought were important for all persons. So we directly assessed these skills for all the individuals we served and repeated this assessment annually. We refer to this as a core skills assessment, and the core skills assessment is used to develop our learning and clinical objectives for each individual.

Core Skills Assessment (CSA)

Any diagnostic evaluations generally taking place prior to an individual are being referred to NECC. We don't use them unless they are part of what is required in reviewing education plan progress and planning for further education plans, but if we are conducting research or there are other reasons for us to do other types of assessments, we certainly will, but diagnostic evaluations are typically provided by parties outside of NECC.

We feel our core skill assessment (CSA; Dickson et al., 2014) is important from the perspective of giving us a tool for identifying the skills we need to teach and how to target those skills. Dickson et al. conducted a social validation study of our CSA, telling us whether or not other care providers—other professionals—think that the skills that we are targeting are relevant for the population that we are serving. So we're looking to identify foundational skills and we're interested in hierarchically ordering them. The goal of instruction is then to work the individual through those until they acquire them, and then we move on to the next skill. The CSA is an observational analysis geared toward hitting what you might refer to as behavioral cusps or foundational skills.

What are the skill domains that we look at with our core skills assessment? There are discrimination skills—discrimination, from the perspective of those that have not been well immersed in the stimulus control literature (see Sidman, 1994), underlies all symbolic functioning, not just communication, but so much of what we do in the presence of others and in the absence of others. So we assess discrimination skills, verbal behavior, social behavior, self-help skills, health and safety, physical education, and skills needed to demonstrate independence in the community. Our Autism Curriculum Encyclopedia®, see below, is something that you can find online and learn more about at http://acenecc.org/. Beyond the CSA (i.e., if the child has all the those foundational skills), there is an extended scope and sequence that moves from those more rudimentary skills to those that are more appropriate in late elementary and secondary education. With both of these assessments, we have curricula that can be individualized for targeting each of those skills.

Autism Curriculum Encyclopedia®

The ACE® curricula are modifiable in terms of the teaching procedures that one can use dependent on the teaching procedures effective for that individual (see, e.g., Seaver & Bourret, 2014). Establishing an understanding of proper support and motivation for each learner is important, and at NECC we work with what the individual's motivation by assessing preferences and constructing motivational supports as needed. We feel very strongly that preference assessment is only the beginning point in determining whether or not you have effective reinforcers. It is something that needs to be done for each person and, oftentimes, needs to be adjusted with different skills because what's reinforcing in one context is not necessarily reinforcing in another context, just as what is reinforcing for one person's behaviors is not necessarily reinforcing for another person's behavior. Establishing motivational systems based upon that foundational work aids greatly in making consistent progress. Certainly motivational systems exist within the typical environment and that is where we need to get each person eventually, rather than persistent reliance on token economies.

So in terms of what we have within the curriculum, we have multiple teaching strategies that are available, not only discrete trial training, incidental teaching, and modalities of teaching that involve other modeling skills both in vivo and video modeling. The ACE® also has mastery criteria, and we aim to determine whether or not those skills have generalized into the environments in which they need to occur. The CSA is readministered on an annual basis for reviewing progress and setting up our objects going forward from that point. The end goal is independent functioning in the community.

The ACE® requires experience in ABA. For those who are special educators, having regular consultative interaction with those that are experts in ABA is probably necessary to optimize the outcomes using this tool. It is very good for the individual who is overseeing the implementation of ACE-guided instruction to have extensive experience in teaching skills and staff training as well. Currently, there are over 3500 users of the ACE® in 21 states in the United States and nine countries. The cost is about $50 per student per month and there are discounts for large numbers of students. Initially, as a start-up it is a $1200 package that comes with expert guidance, and there is ongoing consultation as one is receiving the ACE® and implementing with those students that they targeted to implement with. It is being used in both public and private schools.

Severe Problem Behavior

As mentioned previously functional analysis is well established within the research literature of applied behavior analysis as a gold standard and function-based interventions are, as well. Certainly in the history of applied behavior analysis, the clinical approach to treatment has always been that the least restrictive yet effective is the most desirable. When it comes to being effective, this least restrictive yet effective does not rule "aversive" out. It is social contingencies that establish what we can and cannot do. I'm going to give an example of what I feel is a way of getting to an innovative, yet effective, least restrictive approach. As I mentioned before, NECC heavily focuses on functional replacement behavior. We also do not use painful aversive procedures, and there are special considerations or expertise that is necessary for more than your garden-variety problem behavior. These are beyond the scope of this piece.

To provide some example, however, repetitive behavior is often automatically maintained (Ahearn, Clark, MacDonald, & Chung, 2007), and thus we don't have access to the contingency maintaining problem behavior. So special considerations, as discussed below, are necessary. Also, when we have medical or dental procedures that need to be conducted and the individual has difficulties with such procedures or they are anxious in a social context, still other atypical interventions strategies, such as systematic desensitization, are necessary.

Staff Skills and Training

So we were also asked to discuss staff skill and training. At NECC all of our direct care staff, which we refer to as teachers, come in through the door with a bachelor's degree. We prefer our frontline supervisors, those that are there on a moment-to-moment basis, to be matriculating through one of our masters programs, either our masters in special education or our masters in applied behavior analysis—the first offered through Simmons College and the second offered through Western New England University, with that program being headed by Rachel Thompson. Moreover we provide extensive training before someone becomes a supervisor. I am going to quantify that below. The managers of caseloads, which we refer to as a program specialist, must have an MA or an MS and their BCBA. We have about 150 BCBAs on staff, and we refer to our supervisors of the program specialists as program directors. They, as a minimum, have 5 years of experience and a minimum of an MA, an MS, and a BCBA with most of them having a PhD in applied behavior analysis or a human service profession.

What does NECC provide in terms of training? In consultation with NECC's director of training, Allen Karsina, he quantified the number of training opportunities as the grossest measure that we have of training. He estimated that there are 1000 training opportunities per year per staff member that are occurring for our staff. Our direct care staff, in terms of those things that we sort, pull out and are looking more specifically in terms of observing performance; there are 100+ hours that we provide in training before the individual starts to work with students. There are weekly team meetings, quarterly trainings, and refreshers, plus several other annual trainings that add up to 1000 training opportunities per year. In addition, there are 90-day evaluations and annual evaluations that are performed for all staff. Our supervisors, in addition to having those trainings, there is a minimum of 24 additional hours in supervisor training annually that they are required to have, in addition to whatever continuing education is necessary to maintain their certification and/or licensure.

An Overview of the Approach

In terms of an overview of the NECC approach or the evidence base for our model, the way I like to characterize this is the NECC way—using research to inform best practice. And what does best practice mean? That is an excellent question to be asked because we use that term "best practice," and I think there are as many times that we use the term "best practice" as there are meanings to the term. That said, when we assert something is a best practice, when there is single-subject research into the teaching procedures and treating excessive behavior that are shown to be effective for those things, we are targeting that this is the frontline of best practice. That is how we determine whether or not we found that there is something that has produced marked, believable change for an individual as a starting point, but it is only a starting point because our questions then is, "what is the best procedure for that individual and for the presenting problem that we have?" So to further lay out what I mean when I say best practice, this is only the tip of the iceberg.

Stages of best practice start with what we do know that is effective and works, but there are oftentimes many different things that work. For instance, we talk about training vocal imitation skills. We know that the direct reinforcement of imitating a vocalization is often effective (e.g., Baer, Peterson, & Sherman, 1967). One models the response and reinforces imitating it directly, but that does not always work. Sundberg, Michael, Partington, and Sundberg (1996) demonstrated a different procedure, referred to as stimulus-stimulus pairing, as a way to bring about vocal imitation. That does not always work either. There is another procedure (Drash, High, & Tudor, 1999), the Mand-Model, which has also been used to establish vocal imitations skills. That does not always work either, but once we identify all those different things that work, what we can do is a comparative study. We compare them to one another to see if there is a most effective procedure. Oftentimes, there is not necessarily one procedure that is universally effective; rather, there are clusterings of individuals that benefit from each procedure. We identify what the characteristics of the learners that respond to each intervention and use those to identify what will likely be effective with the students we are now targeting to teach those skills to.

The Evidence Base

So, what is that evidence base? What would I put out there as some of the most important studies? Well, definitely the early Lovaas studies (Lovaas, 1987, 1996; McEachin, Smith, & Lovaas, 1993) were critically important for establishing that applied behavior analysis is an effective technique. I also included as critically important the recent

Howard et al. studies (2005, 2014) that show that early intensive behavioral intervention applied from a pure applied behavior analytic standpoint is much more effective than an eclectic approach and much more effective than an eclectic intensive approach. Other things that I think are particularly important include meta-analyses. One of the, I think, best studies is by Eldevik et al. (2009), showing that early intensive behavioral intervention produces large significant gains in adaptive behavior and moderate significant gains in behavioral excesses. In addition to that, there is the Cochrane review that was published by Reichow, Barton, Boyd, and Hume (2012) suggesting ABA as effective for young children with autism though the review also notes that further research is necessary.

Very recently another important study is one that more specifically talks about our model of service delivery. MacDonald, Parry-Cruwys, Dupere, and Ahearn (2014), published in *Research in Developmental Disabilities*, is a study looking at children receiving early intensive behavioral intervention through NECC. This study concentrated on children younger than three and looking at what are possible predictors of outcome from EIBI. The best predictor of outcome, in terms of cognitive performance, was something that was a little surprising to us and that was age. Those that entered early intensive behavioral intervention at 18–23 months of age improved most. What do I mean by improved the most? All those children regardless of whether they initially were rated as low, middle, or high in cognitive score all ended up in the high cognitive score category after EIBI. Early is better, but then again that has long been presumed evident. In terms of cognitive performance on intake and the change you see at exit, there was a marked change for all of the age groups studied with there being an optimal level of change for those individuals entering ABA between 18 and 23 months.

MacDonald, Parry-Cruwys, Dupere, & Ahearn (2014; RIDD)

Table 5. Statistical comparisons across outcome measures and age groups

	RJA Point	RJA Gaze	IJA	Cognitive	Play
Main Effect (Time)	$F(1, 91)=15.14, p<.01$	$F(1, 91)=25.14, p<.01$	$F(1, 91)=4.06, p<.01$	$F(1, 91)= 24.57, p<.01$	$F(1, 91)=7.92 p<.01$
Main Effect (Age)	$F(1, 91)=23.12, p<.01$	$F(3, 91)=3.66, p>.01$	$F(3, 91)=8.50, p<.01$	$F(3, 91)=1.66, p>.01$	$F(3, 91)=4.36, p>.01$
Interaction	$F(1, 91)=12.14, p<.01$	$F(3, 91)=2.54, p>.01$	$F(3, 91)=7.50, p<.01$	$F(3,91)=12.87, p<.01$	$F(3, 91)=14.36, p<.01$
Post-hoc tests	18-23-month-olds improved more than all other age groups; no differences between other age groups	N/A (Scores increased from Time 1 to Time 2)	18-23-month-olds improved more than all other age groups; no differences between other age groups	18-23-month-olds improved more than all other age groups. 24-30-month-olds group improved more than 2.5 and 3-year-olds	18-23-month-olds improved more than all other age groups; no differences between other age groups

Outcome Analysis – Cognitive Performance by Age

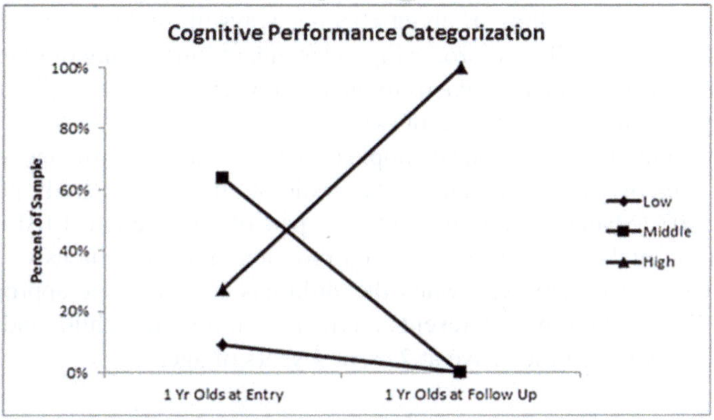

The New England Center for Children®
A leader in autism research and education

Outcome Analysis – Cognitive Performance

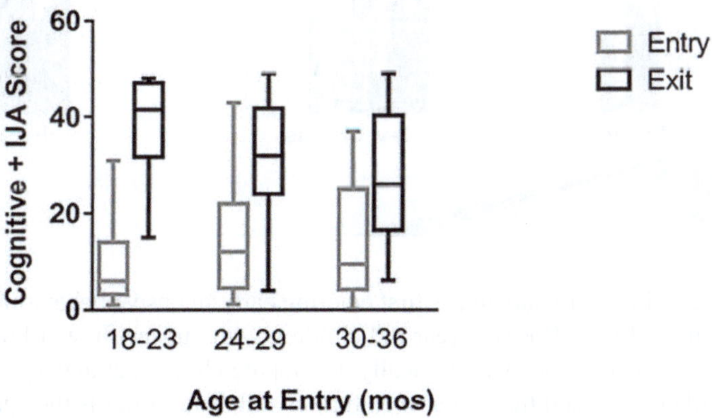

The New England Center for Children®
A leader in autism research and education

So, applied behavior analysis. What do we now know? In terms of the status of the evidence that is out there, we know that behavior analysis, when it is applied effectively, works. That said more work is necessary to identify effective treatments for all of our behavioral objectives. In terms of skill building, we have an awful lot of that inductive data, telling us about effective ways of establishing verbal behavior, play, and social skills and producing independent functioning or outcomes. But more research is necessary to take us to the point where we have empirically identified the best practices in each area of skill.

I'm now going to provide one example of how we have identified a best practice at NECC. Stereotypy is a crucial characteristic of autism. In a study published in RIDD in 2007 (MacDonald et al., 2007), as part of the standard EIBI assessment conducted on intake into our home-based program and early intensive instruction program, we assess stereotypy when the child has access to age-appropriate play materials. Each yellow bar represents a typically developing child, and this is the level of stereotypy that they have at 2, 3, or 4 years of age.

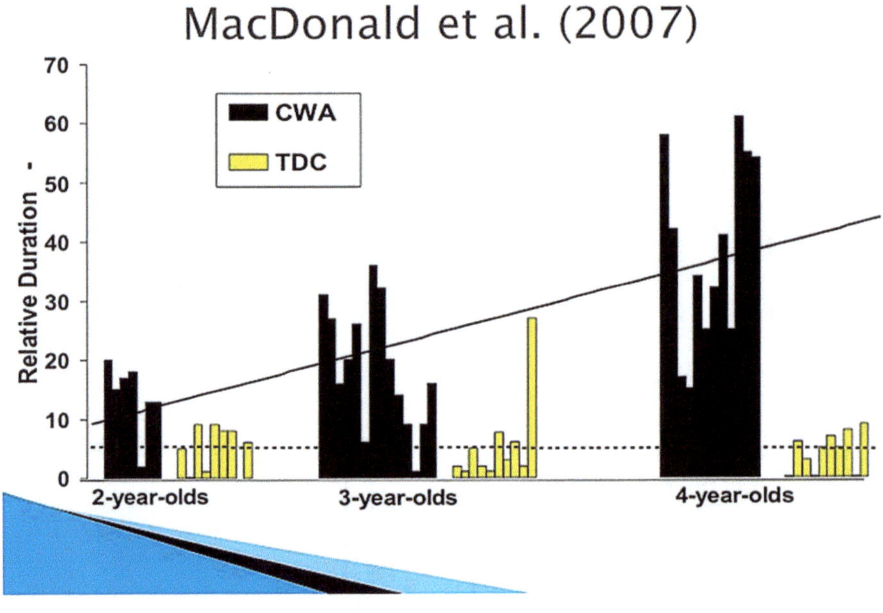

So children with autism are first entering early intensive behavioral intervention at the indicated age. The two-year-old children with autism show a level of stereotypy near that which we see with typically developing children at that age. The 3-year-olds are further away and the 4-year-olds further still. The earlier is the age at which intervention occurs, the closer the child is to their typical peers. Is any individual born with repetitive behavior? They certainly are. We see this in both typically developing and atypically developing individuals, but what happens with children with autism is they are learning. They're learning to recruit reinforcers to produce those stimuli that they prefer to be in the presence of or that make the environment less aversive.

From a behavior analytic perspective, one could conceptualize autism as a social learning disorder (Ahearn, Parry-Cruwys, Toran, & MacDonald, 2015). People with autism are born differently. They are born differently, and attending to different stimuli in different ways and their learning is trapped by or stuck to those stimuli that are most relevant to them. People with autism seem to prefer sensory consequences relative to social consequences. Typically developing people have a general preference for social consequences. Stereotypy produces sensory consequences, and for this reason we tend to see much more stereotypy in persons with autism. When stereotypic behavior is occurring in the presence of other people, it can be problematic. Typically developing people engaging in stereotypic behavior eventually contact social consequences that makes it less likely to occur, while autistic individuals may be more influenced by the sensory consequence. (As an aside however, if one engages in stereotypic behavior and prefers it, and it is not harmful to them or other people, then there should be some time in the day in which it is okay to engage in this type of behavior.) Stereotypy is oftentimes interfering in an instructional context or when we're attempting to provide opportunities to socially interact. So that is why it is often necessary to treat stereotypy. So when we started our investigations into improving procedures for addressing stereotypic responding, we reviewed the literature.

There were many manualized recommendations that seemed like they made good sense and provided a starting point. They tended to recommend redirecting stereotypic behavior but the status of the empirical evidence was very poor. There were also a number of case reports in the behavior analytic literature showing that response blocking for automatically reinforced self-injurious behavior was a pretty effective approach (e.g., Lerman & Iwata, 1996; Smith, Russo, & Le, 1999). Therefore we started with what we thought would be a critical treatment component, response interruption and redirection (RIRD; Ahearn et al., 2007).

RIRD is fairly straightforward of an approach, and in our initial baseline, we don't interact with the individual, providing the motivational conditions most likely to produce stereotypic behavior. If the student did something appropriate, we responded to it with a naturalistic consequence During treatment, contingent upon vocal stereotypy, we established the attention of the individual, and we asked them questions that they knew the answer to and readily complied with such as: "What's your name?" "Where do you live?" "How many licks does it take to get to the center of a Tootsie Pop?" Each of the questions asked was very strongly established within their repertoire. That is, they could perform these tasks, and, of course, if they were behaving appropriately, we would respond with a natural appropriate consequence.

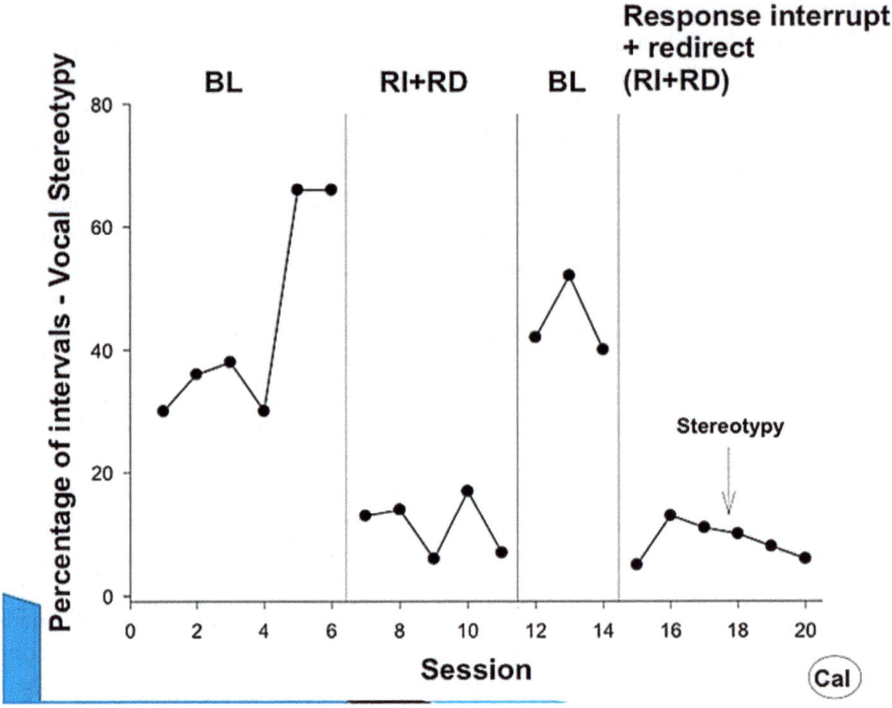
Response interrupt
+ redirect
(RI+RD)
BL
RI+RD
BL
Percentage of intervals - Vocal Stereotypy
80
60
40
20
0
Stereotypy
0
2
4
6
8
10
12
14
16
18
20
Session
Cal

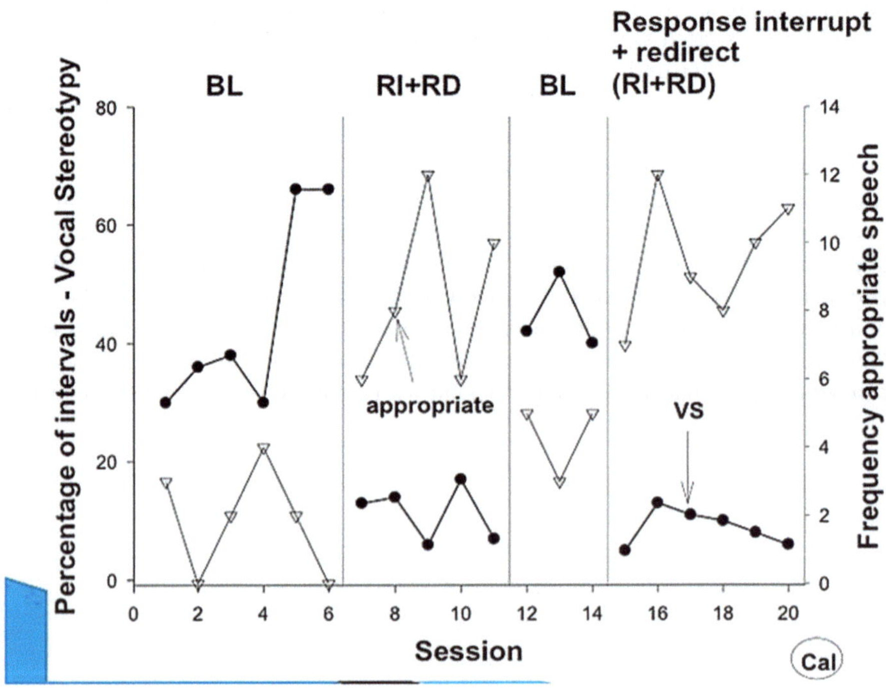
Response interrupt
+ redirect
(RI+RD)
BL
RI+RD
BL
Percentage of intervals - Vocal Stereotypy
80
60
40
20
0
appropriate
VS
Frequency appropriate speech
14
12
10
8
6
4
2
0
0
2
4
6
8
10
12
14
16
18
20
Session
Cal

In this first study, we have four individuals where we had a very quick decrease in the stereotypic behavior and a concomitant increase in appropriate vocalizations with three of the four students. This study spurred a flurry of single-subject studies on this particular technique, nicely reviewed by Martinez and Betz in 2013 in the *Journal of Applied Behavior Analysis*. They note that several variants in the response interruption and redirection technique were effective and treatment comparisons generally favor RIRD. However, as I alluded to the above, no one intervention is ever universally effective. It is also the case that added components that target supporting adaptive skills are likely superior to RIRD alone, as we showed in Colón, Ahearn, Clark, and Masalsky (2012).

One could certainly state that this is just a bunch of single-subject studies. However, Vanderkerken and colleagues (2013) conducted a meta-analysis of what they refer to as single-case experiments for vocally challenging behavior, where they looked at 74 cases with a very large treatment effect being found in meta-analysis for procedures like RIRD, with the largest effects being produced by interventions that combined antecedent and consequent interventions, as in Colón et al. (2012). Thus, we have, in fact, best practice evidence that brings to scale the knowledge that allows us to more effectively intervene with individuals as we encounter them with that particular presentation.

Establishing appropriate behavior is very important. When we teach social interaction (and sometimes it is as simple as using prompting to get the behavior to occur) or when we teach play skills via prompting or with whatever necessary supports that need to be there to get it to occur, oftentimes the collateral effect is that we see less stereotypy. So at the New England Center for Children, our approach is this type of research to practice approach, and, oftentimes, what we get when we use research to drive our practices is that we then encounter questions as we go along in our practice that better informs the next research study we are doing. So when setting our goals as clinicians, research can help set out our agenda, and for individuals with autism, the goal is very clear, but how to get there is not always clear, but evidence is emerging and emerging very rapidly from a number of sources, not just applied behavior analysts. Research and treatment settings, however, I would say regardless of your orientation, are the best way to identify effective treatment, and these effective teaching tools can be bettered, and by that I mean through research and through research, best practices can be revealed.

References

Ahearn, W. H., Clark, K. M., MacDonald, R. P. F., & Chung, B. I. (2007). Assessing and treating vocal stereotypy in children with autism. *Journal of Applied Behavior Analysis, 40*, 263–275.

Ahearn, W. H., Parry-Cruwys, D., Toran, T., & MacDonald, J. (2015). Stimulus salience in autism: A social learning disorder. In F. DiGennaro Reed (Ed.), *Bridging the gap between science and practice in autism service delivery*. New York: Springer.

Ahearn, W. H., & Tiger, J. H. (2012). Behavioral approaches to the treatment of autism. In G. Madden (Ed.), *APA handbook of behavior analysis, Vol. 2: Translating principles into practice*. Washington, DC: American Psychological Association.

Baer, D. M., Peterson, R. F., & Sherman, J. A. (1967). The development of imitation by reinforcing behavioral similarity to a model. *Journal of the Experimental Analysis of Behavior, 21*, 405–416.

Colón, C. L., Ahearn, W. H., Clark, K. M., & Masalsky, J. (2012). The effects of verbal operant training and response interruption and redirection on appropriate and inappropriate vocalizations. *Journal of Applied Behavior Analysis, 45*(1), 107–120.

Dickson, C. A., MacDonald, R. P. F., Mansfield, R., Guilhardi, P., Johnson, C., & Ahearn, W. H. (2014). Social validation of the New England Center for Children—Core skills assessment. *Journal of Autism and Developmental Disorders, 44*, 65–74.

Drash, P., High, R. L., & Tudor, R. M. (1999). Using mand training to establish an echoic repertoire in young children with autism. *The Analysis of Verbal Behavior, 16*, 29–44.

Eldevik, S., Hastings, R. P., Hughes, J. C., Jahr, E., Eikeseth, S., & Cross, S. (2009). Meta-analysis of early intensive behavioral intervention for children with autism. *Journal of Clinical Child & Adolescent Psychology, 38*(3), 439–450.

Hanley, G. P., Iwata, B. A., & McCord, B. E. (2003). Functional analysis of problem behavior: A review. *Journal of Applied Behavior Analysis, 36*, 147–185.

Howard, J., Sparkman, C., Cohen, H., Green, G., & Stanislaw, H. (2005). A comparison of intensive behavior analytic and eclectic treatments for young children with autism. *Research in Developmental Disabilities, 26*, 359–383.

Howard, J. S., Stanislaw, H., Green, G., Sparkman, C. R., & Cohen, H. G. (2014). Comparison of behavior analytic and eclectic early interventions for young children with autism after three years. *Research in Developmental Disabilities, 35*, 3326–3344.

Hull, C. L. (1935). The conflicting psychologies of learning: A way out. *Psychological Review, 42*, 491–516.

Iwata, B. A., Dorsey, M. F., Slifer, K. J. Bauman, K. E., & Richman, G. S. (1994a). Toward a functional analysis of self-injury. *Journal of Applied Behavior Analysis, 27*, 197–209. (Reprinted from *Analysis and Intervention in Developmental Disabilities, 2*, 3–20, 1982).

Iwata, B. A., Pace, G. M., Dorsey, M. F., Zarcone, J. R., Vollmer, T. R., Smith, R. G., … Willis, K. D. (1994b). The functions of self-injurious behavior: An experimental-epidemiological analysis. *Journal of Applied Behavior Analysis, 27*, 215–240

Lerman, D. C., & Iwata, B. A. (1996). A methodology for distinguishing between extinction and punishment effects associated with response blocking. *Journal of Applied Behavior Analysis, 29*, 231–233.

Lovaas, O. I. (1987). Behavioral treatment and normal educational and intellectual functioning in young autistic children. *Journal of Consulting and Clinical Psychology, 55*, 3–9.

Lovaas, O. I. (1996). The UCLA young autism model of service delivery. In C. Maurice, G. Green, & S. C. Luce (Eds.), *Behavioral interventions for young children with autism* (pp. 241–249). Austin, TX: Pro-ed.

MacDonald, R. P. F., Green, G., Mansfield, R. C., Geckeler, A. S., Gardenier, N. C., Anderson, J., … Sanchez., J. (2007). Stereotypy in young children with autism and typically developing children. *Research in Developmental Disabilities, 28*, 266–277.

MacDonald, R., Parry-Cruwys, D., Dupere, S., & Ahearn, W. H. (2014). Assessing progress and outcome of early intensive behavioral intervention for toddlers with autism. *Research in Developmental Disabilities, 35*, 3632–3644.

McEachin, J. J., Smith, T., & Lovaas, O. I. (1993). Long-term outcome for children with autism who received early intensive behavioral treatment. *American Journal on Mental Retardation, 97*, 359–372.

Pelios, L., Morren, J., Tesch, D., & Axelrod, S. (1999). The impact of functional analysis methodology on treatment choice for self-injurious and aggressive behavior. *Journal of Applied Behavior Analysis, 32*, 185–195.

Reichow, B., Barton, E. E., Boyd, B. A., & Hume, K. (2012). Early intensive behavioral intervention (EIBI) for young children with autism spectrum disorders (ASD). *Cochrane Database of Systematic Reviews, 10*, CD009260.

Seaver, J. L., & Bourret, J. C. (2014). An evaluation of response prompts for teaching behavior chains. *Journal of Applied Behavior Analysis, 47*, 777–792.

Sidman, M. (1994). *Equivalence relations and behavior: A research story*. Boston: Authors Cooperative.

Skinner, B. F. (1945). The operational analysis of psychological terms. *Psychological Review, 52*, 270–277.

Skinner, B. F. (1950). Are theories of learning necessary? *Psychological Review, 57*, 193–216.

Skinner, B. F. (1953). *Science and human behavior* (pp. 182–193). New York: The MacMillan Company.

Skinner, B. F. (1957). *Verbal behavior*. New York: Appleton.

Skinner, B. F. (1981). Selection by consequences. *Science, 213*, 501–504.

Smith, R. G., Russo, L., & Le, D. D. (1999). Distinguishing between extinction and punishment effects of response blocking: A replication. *Journal of Applied Behavior Analysis, 32*, 367–370.

Sundberg, M. L., Michael, J., Partington, J. W., & Sundberg, C. A. (1996). The role of automatic reinforcement in early language acquisition. *The Analysis of Verbal Behavior, 13*, 21–37.

Tolman, E. C. (1938). Physiology, psychology, and sociology. *Psychological Review, 45*, 228–241.

Vanderkerken, L., Heyvaert, M., Mayes, B., & Onghena, P. (2013). Psychosocial interventions for reducing vocal challenging behavior in persons with autistic disorder: A multilevel meta-analysis of single-case experiments. *Research in Developmental Disabilities, 34*, 4515–4533. doi:10.1016/j.ridd.2103.09.030.

Watson, J. B. (1913). Psychology as the behaviorist views it. *Psychological Review, 20*, 158–177.

Chapter 5
The Value of a Behavioral Analysis of Language for Autism Treatment

Mark L. Sundberg

Thank you Ron Leaf, Sally Rogers, and Bill Ahearn for your excellent presentations. I've enjoyed listening to you today and learning more about your programs. In general, the message you have all presented so far has been that behaviorally based interventions for children with autism are powerful, and their roots are well-established in the scientific literature. You gave us three examples of what behavior analysis has to offer autism treatment, and I will present a fourth, the applied behavior analysis/verbal behavior (ABA/VB) approach. But first, I would like to acknowledge that what we are collectively presenting here today is just a sample of the many behaviorally based models of autism treatment that are available in the literature. For example, incidental teaching (Hart & Risley, 1975), pivotal response training (Koegel, O'Dell, & Koegel, 1987), and CABAS (Greer & Ross, 2007) all provide solid behavioral intervention programs. These behavioral models, as well as others, all share a common basic foundation in behavior analysis, the branch of psychology initially set forth by B. F. Skinner. The application of behavior analysis to autism treatment has a long and successful history, and because that is the focus of our talks today, I would like to briefly review that history.

History of the Intervention Approach

B. F. Skinner's book *Science and Human Behavior* (1953) is considered to be the conceptual beginning of the field of Applied Behavior Analysis (ABA) (Morris, Smith, & Altus, 2005). The first systematic application of Skinner's analysis of

The author would like to thank Cindy Sundberg for her comments on earlier versions of this chapter.

M.L. Sundberg, Ph.D., B.C.B.A. D. (✉)
Behavior Analysis Center for Autism, Fishers, IN, USA
e-mail: marksundberg@astound.net

R.G. Romanczyk, J. McEachin (eds.), *Comprehensive Models of Autism Spectrum Disorder Treatment*, DOI 10.1007/978-3-319-40904-7_5

behavior to human problems was Ayllon and Michael's (1959) research at Saskatoon State Hospital in Saskatoon, Saskatchewan (Cooper, Heron, & Heward, 2007), where they worked with persons with schizophrenia and/or mental deficiencies. The title of their seminal research paper was "The psychiatric nurse as a behavioral engineer" and was Ayllon's doctoral dissertation at The University of Houston (U of H), with Jack Michael as his advisor. Their research demonstrated the immediate clinical success of several procedures based on operant principles (e.g., reinforcement, extinction, satiation) across a variety of human behaviors (e.g., psychotic talk, excessive entering of the nurses' office, self-feeding, magazine hording). Ferster (1961) provided the first behavioral analysis of the problems faced by children with autism, along with a line of related experimental research (e.g., Ferster & DeMyer, 1962). During that same time period, Sidney Bijou, who was a departmental colleague of Skinner's in the 1940s at Indiana University, was developing applications of Skinner's work at the Institute of Child Development in Seattle, WA. Bijou was a professor at the University of Washington (U-of-W) and the director of the Institute.

Jack Michael and B. F. Skinner, circa 1979

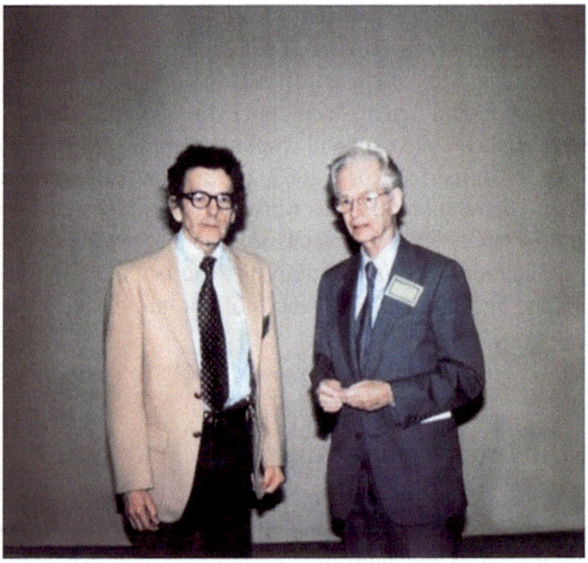

Jack Michael and Ted Ayllon, circa 2008

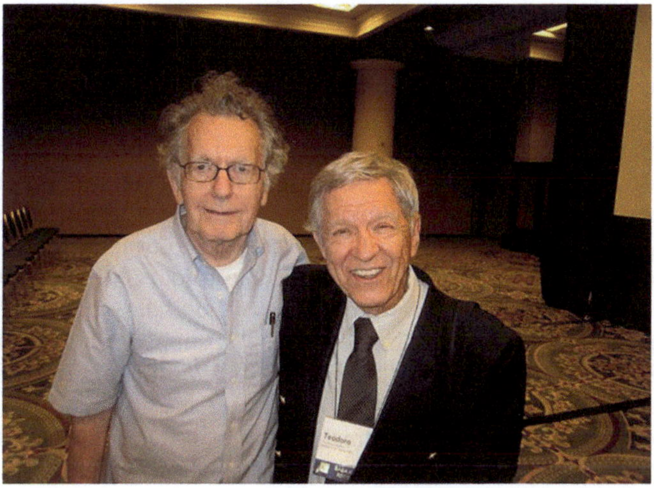

Charles B. Ferster, circa, 1972

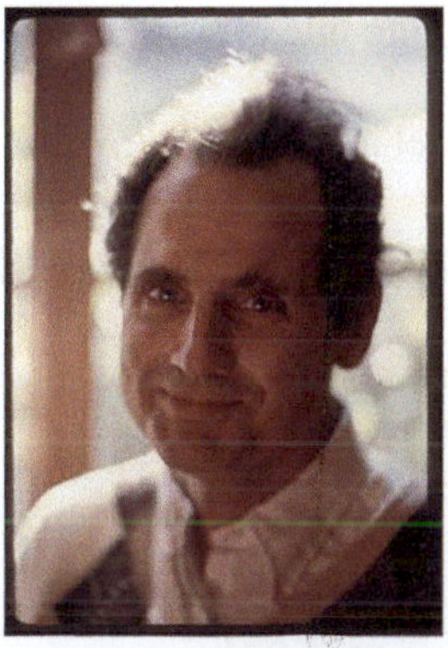

Sidney Bijou, circa, 1990

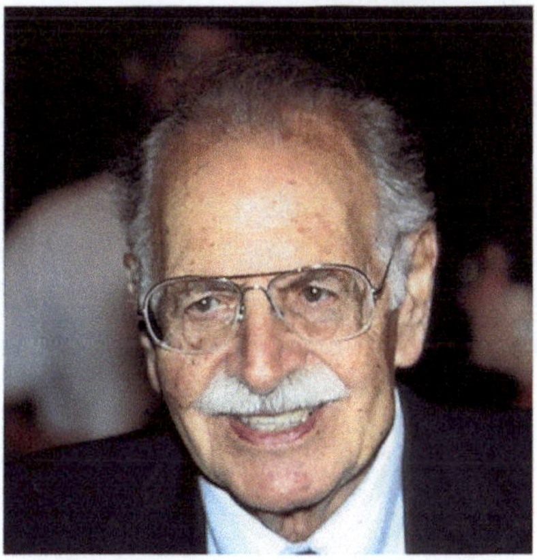

By the late 1950s, Bijou had assembled an impressive team of students and professors at U-of W to work at the Institute. They established the first university-based clinical program that systematically applied behavioral principles and procedures to children with autism or other types of disabilities. Among Bijou's team was a fellow faculty member at U-of-W, Donald Baer. Bijou recruited several others to join them, including one of Jack Michael's Ph.D. students from Arizona State University (ASU), Montrose Wolf. Todd Risley was an undergraduate student at U-of-W at the time and also joined the team. Many of our field's early contributors participated in Bijou's program over the years including Jay Birnbrauer, Barbara Etzel, R. Vance Hall, Betty Hart, Rob Hawkins, Bill Hopkins, Ivar Lovaas, Jim Sherman, and Howard Sloane to name a few. In his memoriam to Bijou, Ghezzi (2010) wrote that this list of participants in Bijou's lab "reads like a who's who of pioneers in behavior analysis" (pp. 176–177). Ghezzi also noted that, "If applied behavior analysis has a birthplace it would be in Seattle at the University of Washington's Institute of Child Development with Sid at the helm" (p. 177). In fact, the first published application of behavioral principles to autism treatment was a study conducted at Bijou's Institute (Wolf, Risley, & Mees, 1964). That study presented many firsts in our field, including the first to use a reversal design, time out, reports of social validity, and the first to describe their intervention strategy as "discrete trial" instruction. Thus, it is quite clear that current models of ABA intervention for children with autism have their roots in this groundbreaking line of work, guided by Sid Bijou.

Jack Michael and Montrose Wolf, circa, 1975

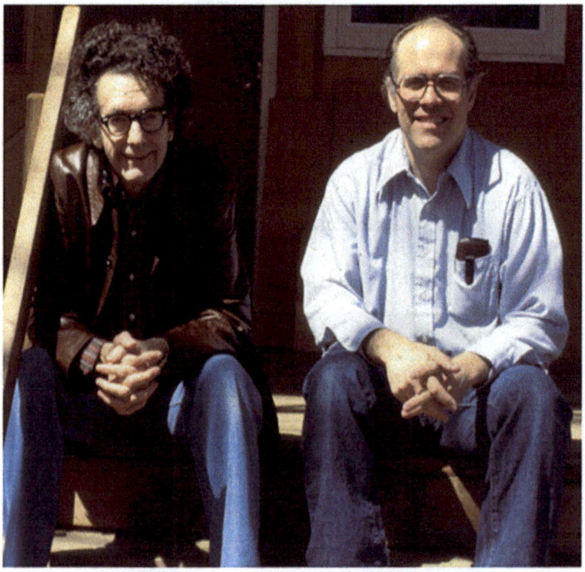

Donald Baer, Montrose Wolf, and Todd Risley, circa, 1999

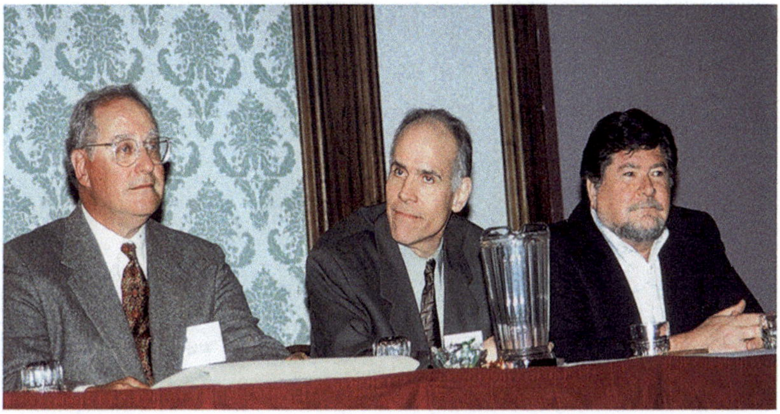

The particular approach to autism treatment that I am going to present, "applied behavior analysis/verbal behavior" (ABA/VB) (also termed the "verbal behavior approach"), has its roots in the same history described above, as well as a history of its own, but involving some of the same pioneers identified above. Skinner published another book in the 1950s titled *Verbal Behavior* (1957). That book elaborated on several issues raised and discussed in *Science and Human Behavior* (1953), but primarily those that involved language. Skinner described a complete behavioral analysis of language that differed so significantly from all other treatments of language at the time that verbal protests erupted (e.g., Chomsky, 1959). Skinner's book was based on the basic principles of behavior and data published from the various animal and human operant research labs operating at the time. Skinner analyzed language as learned behavior under the control of the same environmental contingencies that control nonverbal behavior (i.e., stimulus control, motivation, reinforcement, extinction) and argued against the cognitive theories of language popular at the time. Skinner (1957) termed his approach to language as "A functional analysis of verbal behavior" (p. 1).

Jack Michael is widely recognized for his long-standing contributions to refining, teaching, and disseminating Skinner's analysis of verbal behavior (e.g., Michael, 1982, 1984, 1988, 2004). He began teaching verbal behavior in 1955 using a draft of Skinner's book, and along with his U-of-H and ASU colleague Lee Meyerson, began to undertake applied challenges such as deafness and intellectual disabilities (e.g., Meyerson & Michael, 1964). During that same time period, Joe Spradlin, at the University of Kansas and Parsons State Hospital, developed the first application of Skinner's analysis of verbal behavior to language assessment for low-verbal institutionalized persons (Spradlin, 1963). Spradlin was also instrumental in the early applications of Skinner's work on language to the development of intervention programs for persons with intellectual disabilities (e.g., Spradlin, 1966).

Lee Meyerson, circa, 1974

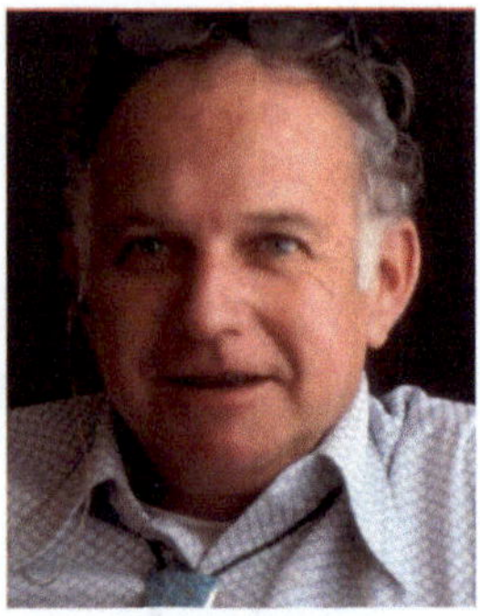

Joseph Spradlin, circa, 1979

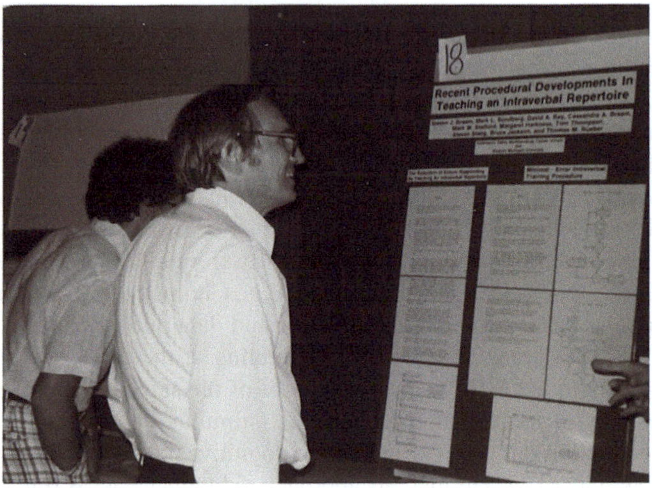

Michael moved to Western Michigan University (WMU) in 1967 where he continued to teach a course on Skinner's analysis of verbal behavior every academic year and eventually added a "verbal behavior applications" course to his list of offerings (Sundberg, Michael, & Peterson, 1977). In addition, Michael was the research advisor for the Kalamazoo Valley Multihandicap Center (KVMC), a school district program directed by Jerry Shook (who later co-founded the Behavior Analyst Certification Board). KVMC provided services for approximately 70 multiply impaired children and young adults and was primarily staffed by WMU psychology department students. I was one of Michael's M.A. and Ph.D. students and the director of research at KVMC. Over a 6-year period during the 1970s, our group conducted approximately 50 research projects on verbal behavior and teaching language to children with disabilities. Many of these projects were theses or dissertations for Michael's students. Most of this research was presented at the early

Midwestern Association for Behavior Analysis and the Association for Behavior Analysis conferences. Several of these studies and projects were eventually published in various behavioral journals and books (e.g., Braam & Poling, 1983; Hall & Sundberg, 1987; Stafford, Sundberg, & Braam, 1988; Sundberg, 1983; Sundberg, Michael, Partington, & Sundberg, 1996; Touchette & Howard, 1984).

Jack Michael, Ivar Lovaas, and Mark Sundberg, circa, 1979

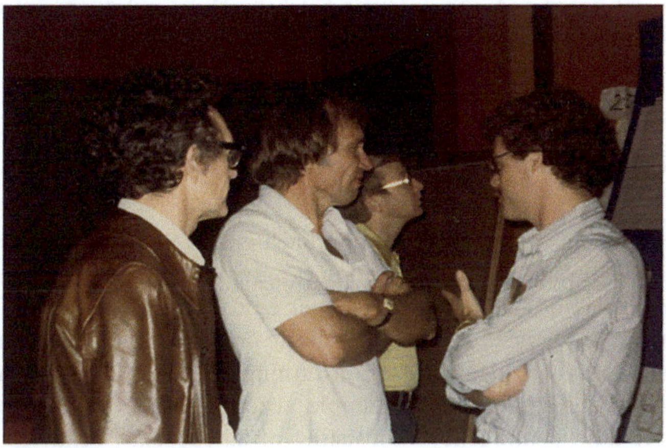

Spradlin's work on a behavioral approach to language assessment provided the foundation for later work on assessment (McGreevy, Fry, & Cornwall, 2012; Partington & Sundberg, 1998; Sundberg, 1983, 2007, 2008, 2014; Sundberg & Partington, 1998), as did his work on language intervention (Sundberg, 1980, 2007; Sundberg & Partington, 1998). As a result of the encouragement of Catania, Day, Glenn, Michael, Skinner, Spradlin, E. Vargas, Wood, and others at an ABA Special Interest Group meeting (Wood & Michael, 1977), I started a verbal behavior newsletter (VB NEWS) that later became the journal *The Analysis of Verbal Behavior* (TAVB). I was the Editor of that journal for the first 14 volumes. Currently, it is published by the Association for Behavior Analysis: International and is in its 32nd volume. Much of the conceptual and empirical basis for the ABA/VB approach can be found among the 352 papers published in TAVB, along with many additional verbal behavior papers published in variety of other journals, books, and online outlets.

Foundational Aspects of the ABA/VB Approach

The ABA/VB approach originated from the work of those cited above, especially B. F. Skinner, Jack Michael, and Joe Spradlin. I am going to suggest four basic components of this approach, all of which are derived from behavior analysis (Table 5.1).

Table 5.1 Four foundational aspects of the ABA/VB approach

1.	The teaching procedures are based on the basic concepts and principles of behavior analysis (e.g., Michael, 2004; Skinner, 1953)
2.	The language assessment and intervention programs are based on Skinner's (1957) analysis of verbal behavior
3.	The target skills and curriculum sequence are based on a behavioral analysis of human development and related research (e.g., Bijou & Baer, 1961, 1965, 1967; Novak & Pelaez, 2004; Schlinger, 1995)
4.	A behavioral analysis of language, learning, and social barriers that can impede progress is ongoing (Sundberg, 2014)

The Concepts and Principles of Behavior Analysis

The first component of the ABA/VB approach is that the specific teaching procedures that make up the daily intervention program are based on the concepts and principles of behavior analysis (e.g., Cooper et al., 2007; Michael, 2004; Skinner, 1953; Sundberg & Michael, 2001). These basic procedures are common to all intervention methods that are identified as constituting a behavioral approach (e.g., DTT, ABA, EIBI, PRT, ABA/VB). For example, teaching trials involve the commonly termed "three-term contingency" consisting of antecedents, behavior, and consequences. In a structured teaching arrangement, if the target is to teach a child to tact a specific item (e.g., a cup), the instructor would present the item while prompting the child to respond with a general verbal prompt (e.g., "What is it?") and possibly with a direct echoic prompt (e.g., "Say cup") and differentially reinforce successive approximations to the target behavior. The instructor would gradually fade out the prompts over a number of teaching trials in order to establish the nonverbal stimulus as a discriminative stimulus (S^D) that evokes the targeted tact response. This is the basic discrete trial teaching (DTT) format that was first introduced by Wolf et al. (1964), elaborated on extensively by Lovaas (1977), and now common in the behavioral treatment of autism (e.g., Maurice, Green, & Luce, 1996).

In a natural environment teaching arrangement (e.g., Hart & Risley, 1975; Koegel et al., 1987), the same three-term-contingency framework also guides the intervention, but this arrangement makes use of a child's motivating operations (MOs), as well as naturally occurring stimuli, routines, and activities in the child's daily environment. For example, if a child initiates an interaction to play with a train set (MO is strong), attempts to establish various forms of stimulus control are implemented. If a particular imitative behavior is desired (e.g., pushing the train), that behavior would be modeled by an adult, who would then prompt the child to imitate her, and if at least an approximation to the target behavior occurs, praise and perhaps other reinforcers are delivered. The ABA/VB approach makes use of both discrete trial teaching and natural environment teaching methods. (For more detail on the distinction between these teaching strategies, related research, and the suggested need for both methodologies, see Sundberg & Partington, 1999.)

Table 5.2 A sample of 25 behavioral principles and concepts

Motivating operations	Stimulus control
Prompting	Fading
Shaping	Chaining
Reinforcement	Extinction
Differential reinforcement procedures (e.g., DRO, DRI)	Pairing
Intermittent reinforcement procedures (e.g., VR, FI, VI)	Modeling
Structured and natural environment teaching methods	Generalization
Transfer of stimulus control techniques	Errorless learning
Behavioral momentum techniques	Fluency procedures
Conditional discrimination training	Task analysis
Contingency contracting	Token economies
Multiple exemplar training	Interspersal methods
Functional and descriptive analyses	

There are hundreds of different teaching procedures that make up an ABA style program. These procedures are based on the concepts and principles of behavior analysis and have many variations (e.g., Cooper et al., 2007; Michael, 2004). A sample of 25 of the basic behavioral principles and concepts is presented in Table 5.2. In the behavioral literature, each of these topics often has its own chapter, or even an entire book devoted to it (e.g., *The Token Economy*, by Ayllon & Azrin, 1968). A primary task for those who design and implement ABA programs is to teach staff and parents how to implement behavioral procedures, as well as how to determine when a procedure is appropriate for a given problem or child. More details on the scientific background, technical concepts, procedures, and methodology of applied behavior analysis can be found in any one of a number of textbooks currently available (e.g., Cooper et al., 2007; Malott & Shane, 2013; Martin & Pear, 2015; Miltenberger, 2015; Sulzer-Azaroff, Mayer, & Wallace, 2013).

Skinner's (1957) Analysis of Verbal Behavior

The second component of ABA/VB, the application of Skinner's (1957) analysis of verbal behavior, is the most distinguishing aspect of the ABA/VB approach. Given that "social communication" deficits constitute the primary diagnostic criteria for autism according to the DSM-5, any approach for teaching children with autism should contain an intensive language intervention component. The question is what theory of language should be used to frame the assessment and intervention process? There are many choices with the majority of views stemming from biological or cognitive theories of language (e.g., Brown, 1973; Bruner, 1983; Chomsky, 1957; McNeill, 1970; Piaget, 1952; Pinker, 1994; Slobin, 1973). Noam Chomsky stands out as one of the most famous psycholinguists, perhaps best known for his strong criticism of Skinner's analysis of verbal behavior (Chomsky, 1959). But, despite the commonly held (and erroneous) view that Chomsky proved Skinner and his views of language wrong, behavioral psychology, including Skinner's analysis of verbal behavior, provides the core of modern day "effective-treatments" for children with autism (National Standards Project, 2014). On the other hand, there is to date no known application of Chomsky's theory to autism treatment offered by those who maintain Chomsky's position on language acquisition.

However, cognitive psychology still provides the foundation for most language assessment and intervention programs used for children with autism (Esch, LaLonde, & Esch, 2010). In this traditional conceptual framework of language, it is characteristic to divide language into expressive and receptive components (e.g., Brown, 1973). Skinner (1957) argued against this dichotomy and conceptual foundation of language for a number of reasons. Perhaps most relevant to our goals of teaching children with autism to communicate is that "expressive language" is actually comprised of several different language functions. That is, the same word can have different functions (or "meanings"), and a child with autism may demonstrate one function of a word, but not another. For example, a child could say "spoon" because he sees a spoon (called a "tact" by Skinner), or he could say "spoon," because he needs a spoon and none are present ("mand"), or he could say "spoon" when none are visible, but he hears "knife, fork, and…" (intraverbal). From Skinner's point of view, despite that the same word is emitted in each example, that word is evoked by different antecedents, and thus have different functions. It is not uncommon to identify children with autism who can emit one function (often tacting) but not the others. Thus, when one term "expressive language" is applied to all three of these different functions, important distinctions and possible language deficits can be missed in the assessment and intervention process.

I would like to offer a quote from Skinner (1957), early in his book *Verbal Behavior*: "What happens when a [person] speaks or responds to speech is clearly a question about human behavior and hence a question to be answered with the concepts and techniques of psychology as an experimental science of behavior." (p. 5). So, early on in the book, Skinner makes his position clear: language is behavior. Thus, behavior analysis should participate in the analysis and understanding of this type of behavior. He also states, "we don't find this field unoccupied" (p. 3). We are not the first ones to offer an analysis of language, but Skinner's basic and unique premise is that speaking and listening constitute behavior. So if they are behaviors, they are a function of antecedents and consequences, and a specific learning history, just like nonverbal behavior. Thus, from Skinner's point of view, the same basic principles of behavior that apply to nonverbal behavior (e.g., stimulus control, MOs, reinforcement, extinction) also apply to verbal behavior. There are no new principles of behavior required to explain language. The only difference between the two is in the way they are reinforced. Nonverbal behavior obtains its reinforcement directly from the environment, whereas verbal behavior obtains its reinforcement through the behavior of another person, that is, it is a socially mediated type of reinforcement, and a complete verbal episode involves both a speaker and a listener (for more detail on the definition of verbal behavior see Normand, 2009).

Earlier, Bill Ahearn talked about the difference between functional and structural approaches to understanding human behavior. For the most part, autism treatment is dominated by structural approaches to language. Bill pointed out some of the problems of structural approaches to working with behavior problems and the clear advantages, clinically, for using a functional approach. For example, if one is asked to work with a child who pulls others' hair, the structural quantification of hair pulling alone will not identify the cause of the behavior, which is what the clinician needs to know in order to change the behavior. The behavior analyst would look at a negative behavior like hair pulling and ask, "What's the function?" "What's the source of control for this behavior?" "What are the antecedents that evoke the behavior?" "What are the consequences?" "What is the history of this behavior?" "Is the behavior related to motivating operations or verbal behavior?" Knowing the function of a behavior tells us what to do. The same problems that Bill identified for structural approaches to behavior problems exist for structural approaches to language. What is most important is not the specific words that are emitted, but the sources of control that evoke these words, that is, the relevant antecedents, consequences, and learning history. A functional analysis is the basis of behavior analysis, including Skinner's analysis of language.

The field of speech and language pathology and applied behavior analysis share much in common when it comes to the treatment of children with autism. I've worked in many different public schools, private schools, and homes over the years, and speech and language pathologists (SLPs) are often on the same page as behavior analysts. We may have different terms and talk differently about language, but our goals are often the same. We have to teach the child to communicate. We have to teach him to request (or mand for) the things he wants using words, signs, or icon exchange. We have to teach him to name objects and actions in his environment, understand what those words mean, imitate our actions and words, and so on. SLPs have long used the basic principles and concepts of behavior analysis, that is, they use prompting, fading, shaping, differential reinforcement, etc., as key elements of their intervention procedures. Over the past few decades, however, the field of speech pathology is moving closer and closer to a functional analysis of language, and I think work in the area of autism is facilitating that union.

Support for this transition to a functional analysis of language comes from within the field of speech pathology. Hedge (2010), an author of several speech pathology textbooks notes, "SLPs have successfully used the behavioral intervention procedures….If the SLPs also adopt a functional (cause-effect) analysis of verbal behaviors, they would then be internally more consistent with their concepts and treatment methods. Treatment research in child language disorders has generally supported Skinner's view that verbal behavior is not organized structurally, but functionally" (p. 110). However, structural approaches to language still dominate language assessment and intervention programs for children with autism. While Skinner's analysis of verbal behavior was published 60 years ago, the basic principles of behavior have not changed and his analysis is still quite relevant to the current efforts to teach language to persons in whom it is absent or impaired.

Skinner (1957) preferred the terms "speaker" and "listener" over the terms "expressive language" and "receptive language" for a number of reasons. Perhaps most bothersome to Skinner was that in traditional cognitive theories of language "Common processes are suggested when language is said to arouse in the mind of the listener 'ideas present in the mind of the speaker,' or when communication is regarded as successful only if an expression has 'the same meaning for both speaker and listener.' Theories of meaning are usually applied to both speaker and listener as if the meaning process were the same for both" (pp. 34–35).

Skinner's Analysis of Speaker Behavior

The basic premise of Skinner's analysis of verbal behavior is that language constitutes learned behavior under the functional control of environmental contingencies. An important aspect of this analysis is that the same behavior (e.g., saying "spoon" or pulling hair) can have different functions, thus constitute different operant behaviors. In addition, Skinner points out that the speaker and listener have different roles in verbal discourse and must be analyzed separately. Although some important aspects of listening are actually covert speaking (e.g., "thinking") and constitute verbal behavior, that should be analyzed as such (Schlinger, 2008). At the core of Skinner's functional analysis of speaker behavior is the distinction between the mand, tact, and intraverbal (listener behavior is also important and I'll discuss that in more detail shortly). As mentioned previously, these three types of verbal behavior are traditionally all classified in one category, expressive language. Skinner suggests that the expressive classification system lumps together important distinctions between functionally independent types of language. In addition to these three core verbal operants, Skinner (1957) also presents the echoic (including motor imitation as it relates to sign language), textual, transcriptive, and copying-a-text relations. These "elementary verbal operants" are viewed as separate functional units that serve as the basis for building more advanced verbal skills (Michael, Palmer, & Sundberg, 2011). Let us now look more closely at the mand, tact, and intraverbal, and the different sources of control that define these types of verbal behavior.

Mand. The mand is a type of verbal behavior where words (or signs, icon exchanges, etc.) are under the functional control of MOs affecting a speaker. That is, a speaker emits words to ask for things or actions that he wants or does not want. For example, a child may ask for milk that is missing when he needs milk for his cereal. The MO related to eating the cereal and the missing milk primarily controls the mand "milk." The reinforcement for the mand is what Skinner calls "specific reinforcement," in that the response identifies the motivator and the consequence is specific to that motivator and satisfies it (the child gets the milk). The same child may also ask for "up" when he is finished eating and wants to get out of a high chair (a mand regarding removing an aversive). Skinner (1957) coined the term mand because it is conveniently brief and is similar to the common English words "com**mand**," "de**mand**," "repri**mand**," and "**mand**atory."

Mands are very important for the early development of language and for the day-to-day verbal interactions with others. Mands are usually the first type of communication acquired by an infant (Bijou & Baer, 1965; Novak & Pelaez, 2004; Schlinger, 1995; Skinner, 1957). These early mands occur in the form of differential crying or eye contact when an infant is hungry, tired, in pain, cold, afraid, or wants social attention. As the infant grows, crying and eye contact can also occur as a mand for toys, help, movement of objects and people, or for the removal of aversive stimuli. Typically, developing children learn to replace crying with words or other standard forms of communication. Manding lets children interact with others in their world and begins to establish the speaker and listener roles that are essential for further verbal development.

Skinner (1957) points out that the mand is the only type of verbal behavior that "directly benefits the speaker" (p. 36), meaning the mand (often) gets the speaker what he wants such as edibles, toys, activities, attention, or the removal of aversive stimuli. As a result, mands can become strong forms of verbal behavior because they satisfy the needs experienced by the child. Young children often engage in a high rate of manding because of these special effects. Eventually, a child learns to mand for many different reinforcers, including mands for verbal information with words like "what," "who," and "where," and the child's acquisition of new verbal behavior accelerates rapidly (Brown, Cazden, & Bellugi, 1969). Ultimately, mands become quite complex and play a critical role in social interaction, conversations, academic behavior, employment, and virtually every aspect of human behavior. Perhaps one of the most valuable pieces of information about a child with autism is the nature of his existing mand repertoire. Given the role of the mand in typical language development, and its frequent relation to problem behavior (e.g., crying, tantrums, refusal) when a child cannot communicate his needs and wants, many clinical issues can be revealed by an analysis of a child's current ability to mand.

Tact. The tact is a type of language where a speaker verbally identifies items, actions, attributes, locations, relationships, etc. in the immediate physical environment. The speaker has direct contact with these "nonverbal" stimuli through any of his sense modes. For example, if a child says "Dog" because he sees a dog, this type of verbal behavior would be classified as a tact. Skinner (1957) selected the term tact because it suggests that a speaker is making direct contact with the physical environment. Technically, the tact is a verbal operant under the functional control of a nonverbal S^D and it is followed by generalized conditioned reinforcement. The tact relation is closely synonymous with what is commonly identified as "expressive labeling" in many language training programs for children with language delays (e.g., Lovaas, 2003).

There are many nonverbal stimuli in a child's world that he eventually must learn to tact. Some of the first tacts that children may acquire include family member's names, toys, common household objects, clothing, pets, etc. (e.g., mama, ball, kitty, car, cup, book). Nonverbal stimuli come in many forms. They can be, for example, static (nouns), transitory (verbs), relations between objects (prepositions), properties of objects (adjectives), possession of objects or actions (pronouns), properties of actions (adverbs), and so on. Nonverbal stimuli can be simple like a shoe or complex like a shopping mall. A stimulus configuration can also have multiple nonverbal properties (e.g., color, size, location), and a response may be under the control of those multiple properties, as in the tact, "The black dog jumped up on the table and ate my sandwich." Nonverbal stimuli may be observable (e.g., a car) or unobservable (e.g., pain), subtle (e.g., a wink) or salient (e.g., flashing neon lights), or involve properties common to many different nonverbal stimuli (e.g., size, color). Given the variation and ubiquity of nonverbal stimuli in the physical world, it is no surprise that the tact is a primary topic in the study of language (Skinner, 1957; Sundberg, 2015).

Intraverbal. The intraverbal is a type of language where a speaker verbally responds (including sign language) to the words of others. He also can intraverbally respond to his own words as a type of self-listening (e.g., problem solving). In general, intraverbal behavior involves "talking about" things and activities that are not present. For example, saying "farm" as a result of hearing someone say "Old McDonald had a…" is intraverbal behavior. Answering questions like, "What did you do last night?" or "What's your favorite sport?" is also intraverbal behavior. Intraverbal behavior can involve talking about things and activities when they are present, but this would constitute multiple control and should be analyzed as such (Skinner, 1957). Typically developing children emit a high frequency of intraverbal responses in the form of singing songs, telling stories, describing activities, explaining problems, and so on. Intraverbal responses are also important components of many intellectual behaviors (e.g., when asked, "What does a plant need to grow?" saying "water, soil, and sunshine," or, saying "ten" as a result of hearing "five plus five equals…"). An intraverbal repertoire can become quite massive and complex. Typical adolescents and adults have hundreds of thousands of intraverbal connections in their language repertoires, and they may emit thousands of them every day.

In technical terms, an intraverbal occurs when a verbal S^D evokes a verbal response that does not have point-to-point correspondence with the verbal stimulus (Skinner, 1957). No point-to-point correspondence means the verbal stimulus and the verbal response do not match each other, as they do in the echoic and textual relations. Like all verbal operants (except the mand), the intraverbal produces generalized conditioned reinforcement. For example, in an educational context, the reinforcement for correct answers usually involves some form of generalized conditioned reinforcement such as hearing "right" from a teacher, receiving good grades, or the opportunity to move to the next problem or level.

Many children with autism fail to acquire a functioning intraverbal repertoire. While there are various causes of this, one preventable cause is that the intraverbal relation is not assessed as a separate verbal skill and taught accordingly. It is often assumed that intraverbal skills, like manding, will simply develop from training on tact and listener skills. Often, by the time a child's conversational, social, and verbal skills are identified as weak or impaired, they have developed "barriers" such as prompt dependency, rote responding, or negative behavior. An individual's failure to verbally respond to verbal stimuli may make it hard to develop a functional intraverbal repertoire. Children begin to acquire simple intraverbal behavior following the acquisition of a beginning mand, tact, and listener repertoires. It's important to note that "conversations" are comprised of a combination of the different verbal and listening skills, but none are more critical than the intraverbal. For many children, the emergence of intraverbal behavior can be observed at around the age of two. Many of these early intraverbal relations are quite simple, such as songs, animal sounds, and one- and two-word intraverbal associations and relations (e.g., "Mommy and…"). More complex intraverbal responses, such as answering multiple component questions (e.g., "Why do you wear shoes on your feet?"), may not occur with typically developing children until around 3 or 4 years old (Sundberg & Sundberg, 2011).

Distinctions between the mand, tact, and intraverbal. There are many clinical benefits for making the distinction between the mand, tact, and intraverbal for children with autism. An assessment that respects the distinction between the verbal operants may reveal that one operant is strong, (e.g., tact), while others are weak (e.g., mand, intraverbal). That is, even though a child may be able to tact a spoon when he sees a spoon, that the same child may not be able to mand for the spoon when he needs one, or intraverbally answer the question, "What do you eat cereal with?" when a spoon is not visually present. While the response "spoon" is topographically the same in all three examples, the three repertoires are functionally separate behavioral relations (Skinner, 1957). As previously mentioned, it is quite common and accepted to blend these repertoires together as expressive language and not identify the functional differences. Yet, we often see children, for example, who demonstrate strong tact repertoires, but have weak or absent mand and intraverbal skills regarding the same words. One child I worked with could tact over a dozen different types of dinosaurs, but when his dinosaurs were missing he could not mand "dinosaur." Nor could he say "dinosaur" when asked the intraverbal fill-in, "A stegosaurus is a…", despite that he could easily tact "stegosaurus" when asked to do so.

This problem becomes more apparent when we look at common language assessments used for children with autism (Esch et al., 2010). For example, the expressive section of the *Peabody Picture Vocabulary Test* (Dunn & Dunn, 2007) primarily assesses the tact repertoire and then provides a norm-referenced age equivalent score. If you are told your child has a 2.1 expressive vocabulary, the implication is that his language level is approximately that of a typically developing 2-year-old. Yet, a typically developing 2-year-old is far beyond just being able to tact. A 2-year-old also has an extensive mand repertoire. A 2-year-old emits thousands of words a day, with a high rate of unprompted verbal behavior. A 2-year-old demonstrates observational learning, often learns new words in one or two trials, and generalizes and maintains these new words without formal training. Thus, basing an intervention program on the results of a tact assessment alone may not completely identify a child's linguistic needs. In addition, neglect of the other verbal operants may lead to a premature focus on more advanced tacting such as prepositions, adjectives, and adverbs when the child may not be developmentally ready, and potentially producing rote responding.

Skinner's Analysis of Listener Behavior

Skinner (1957) provides extensive detail regarding the behavior of the listener, including two full chapters mostly devoted to the topic (Chaps. 6 and 7). In addition to noting that much of what is termed "listening" is actually covert verbal behavior and should be analyzed as such (Schlinger, 2008), Skinner identifies four different roles of a listener that can be applied to children with autism.

Listener discriminations. The most familiar role of a listener in ABA programs is his ability to understand the words of a speaker, commonly referred to as "receptive language," or "receptive labeling." That is, when a speaker emits words, does the listener comprehend what is said in some measurable manner? At the simplest level, do verbal stimuli (e.g., "jump") evoke a corresponding nonverbal response (i.e., jumping) on the part of the listener? Does the listener discriminate between verbal stimuli (e.g., "jump" "arms up") as demonstrated by differential behaviors? At a more complex level, when verbal stimuli interact with nonverbal stimuli (e.g., "touch car") does the verbal stimulus alter the evocative effect of the nonverbal stimulus in the form of a conditional discrimination (Saunders & Spradlin, 1989)? Much of our treatment efforts with children who have language delays involve establishing these types of discriminations (i.e., receptive discriminations), but they represent only one type of listener skill, although certainly an important type.

Audience participation. A listener also serves as an audience for a speaker. Skinner devotes a whole chapter in the book *Verbal Behavior* (Chap. 7) to audience control. "An audience, then, is a discriminative stimulus in the presence of which verbal behavior is characteristically reinforced and in the presence of which, therefore, it is characteristically strong" (p. 172). Children with language delays also need to learn to serve this role as an audience for others (e.g., making eye contact, emitting facial expression indicating listening is occurring). Skinner identifies several types of audience control, one of which is that an audience sets the occasion for particular topics of discussion. He notes, "A third function of an audience is to select a subject matter. Listeners differ in the extent to which they reinforce different types of verbal operants and, particularly, various classes of intraverbal responses and tacts. Given a single speaker with a specific history and a specific current situation, the audience will determine not only whether verbal behavior occurs, or the subdivision of the language in which it occurs, but also what types of responses are made and 'what is talked about'" (p. 175). For example, if a child with autism is skilled in a certain video game (e.g., Minecraft), his presence among peers with similar interests can function as an S^D to evoke verbal behavior regarding that particular game. Learning to serve as an audience is an important and appreciated aspect of social behavior.

Mediator of reinforcement. A listener also acknowledges and reinforces a speaker in a number of important ways. He may emit behaviors that increase or maintain verbal interactions such as smiling, nodding, agreeing, and making eye contact when a person talks. In addition, the listener may act upon specific words spoken by another person, for example, opening a door upon hearing "Can you open the door for me?"

Learning to behave in this manner may require specific training for children with autism. This repertoire is not the same as listener discriminations skills. Many children with autism have extensive listener discrimination skills (e.g., they could identify a 1000 different pictures if asked), but they may have problems with looking at speakers, acknowledging and reinforcing speakers, or acting upon what they are saying. For these individuals, it is these various nonverbal behaviors that should become the target for intervention. It is important to note that these listener problems are identified in DSM-5 as nonverbal communication skills.

Emotional responses. Skinner also describes an emotional effect of language, that is, words alone can elicit respondent behaviors (e.g., emotions such as fear and joy). He writes "In the behavior of the listener (or reader)…verbal stimuli evoke responses appropriate to some of the variables which have affected the speaker. These may be conditioned reflexes of the Pavlovian variety or discriminated operants. The listener reacts to the verbal stimulus with conditioned reflexes, usually of an emotional sort" (p. 357). For example, when somebody tells you sad news, genuine respondent behaviors (e.g., tears) along with related operant behaviors that are usually described as empathy ("I'm sorry to hear that") may occur. Part of a listener repertoire involves being emotionally affected by verbal stimuli. Displaying empathy is often a problem for children with autism, and establishing this type of listener behavior may help to facilitate caring, compassion, and other empathetic behaviors.

Applications of Skinner's Analysis of Verbal Behavior

Early in *Verbal Behavior* Skinner makes the point that "The formulation is inherently practical and suggests immediate technological applications at almost every step" (p. 12). Many of the 50 research projects conducted in the 1970s that I mentioned previously were designed to address specific communication problems presented by children and young adults with language delays, and indeed there is an abundant supply of applications and research topics available from Skinner's book (e.g., Sundberg, 1991). Current applications of Skinner's analysis cover a wide variety of language issues and populations (for reviews see Oah & Dickinson, 1989; Sautter & LeBlanc, 2006). In an effort to increase awareness of the value of Skinner's contributions to language intervention, Jack Michael and I published a paper (Sundberg & Michael, 2001) suggesting that Skinner's analysis of language had several specific benefits for children with autism. In doing so, we made the point that Skinner's analysis of verbal behavior is "additive" to the existing ABA style of behavioral programs for autism treatment. I would like to describe some of those additional benefits, as well as a couple of others, and how they could add to a child's program.

Incorporate the mand relation into the program. Most ABA-based early intervention programs for children with autism formally target five core domains: matching-to-sample and sorting, motor imitation, vocal imitation, expressive labeling (tact), and receptive labeling (listener discrimination). Teaching procedures for these core skills were first developed in Bijou's lab, and then elaborated on by Lovaas (1977). In our paper (Sundberg & Michael, 2001), we suggest adding the mand relation to those five core skills, and we identify several advantages for doing so. Those five core skills are still quite important, but it is imperative that a child be able to emit verbal behavior under motivational control, so language becomes useful and functional for the child.

An example of the additive nature of the mand involved a project we conducted at KVMC with deaf teenagers with autism who could tact several items using sign language and identify those same items as a listener, but could not mand for those items when they were needed, but missing (Hall & Sundberg, 1987). For example, one participant who enjoyed instant coffee could tact all the items necessary to make the coffee, identify those items as a listener (via sign language), and even independently make coffee. But when one of the necessary items was missing (e.g., hot water), despite that the participant could tact the item when it was present (S^D control), he could not mand for it when it was missing (MO control). An interrupted chain procedure was used to create an MO, and then a prompting and fading procedure was used to transfer antecedent control from an S^D to an MO (i.e., tact to mand transfer). The conclusion of this research was that the mand can be functionally independent from the tact in language acquisition and may need to be directly trained for some individuals. These data demonstrate the value of adding the mand domain to the group of 5 core skills for language intervention programs for children with autism.

Incorporate MOs into the intervention program. Skinner has always treated motivation as an antecedent variable that is separate from stimulus control (Michael, 1982; 2007; Skinner, 1953; Sundberg, 2013). The example I just presented with the coffee and manding exemplifies that distinction. If you are unfamiliar with MOs, I'd suggest reading Jack Michael's (2007) chapter in Cooper et al. (2007), titled "Motivating operations." Motivation is an important cause of human behavior and many aspects of this principle of behavior can be additive to an ABA program for children with autism. The role of the MO as the primary source of control for manding is now well-appreciated, but there are other applications of the MO principle. For example, the MO can be used as an additional antecedent variable to teach skills such as imitating, tacting, listener discriminations, reading, self-care, play, functional living skills, and social behavior. In fact, for some of these skills, the MO may be quite useful. Self-care offers such an example. If I were to ask you "Why do you bath, brush your teeth, and wear clothes that match?" My guess would be that it could be related to an MO to make a good impression on people, or it might make you automatically feel good, or it might allow you to avoid social punishment for not doing so, all of these involve different behavioral effects. Capturing or creating any of these MOs could play a role in teaching and maintaining self-care skills to individuals with disabilities. There are many potential applications of the MO concept to autism treatment (e.g., Carbone, 2013; Sundberg, 1993, 2013), and the ability to use MOs in intervention programs is a powerful set of clinical skills that can improve the results of a child's program.

Incorporate intraverbal training into the program. As previously mentioned, an intraverbal repertoire is not the same as a mand and tact repertoire, even though the same words might be involved. In addition, the presence of a tact repertoire does not guarantee the presence of an intraverbal repertoire, or vice versa. The example I gave previously regarding the spoon provided a demonstration of this. A child may be able to say "spoon" when he sees a spoon, but not be able to answer the question "What do you eat soup with?" In one of the early studies conducted at KVMC, Braam and Poling (1983) demonstrated this separation with teenagers with autism who could tact, for example, home things and school things, but could not answer questions regarding those items ("Can you name some school things?"), until specific intraverbal training was provided. Intraverbal development occurs with typical children well after early mands and tacts are firmly established, which is usually about 2 years of age (Sundberg & Sundberg, 2011). The intraverbal is perhaps the most difficult of the verbal operants to directly teach due to the complexity of stimuli and responses involved (Axe, 2008; Eikeseth & Smith, 2013). However, it is important to include intraverbal training in a child's program, when they are ready, because it is an essential part of our daily verbal interactions with others (e.g., education, safety, socializing with peers). The concept of the intraverbal, and its applications, demonstrates another additive feature of Skinner's analysis of verbal behavior for autism treatment.

Use the verbal operants as a framework for language assessment. I previously mentioned the work of Spradlin (1963) in developing the *Parsons Language Sample* as a tool for language assessment. Spradlin's assessment contained items for echoic, imitation, mand, tact, and intraverbal skills and sections for speech as well as signed responses. This assessment tool went far beyond other tools available at the time to identify language intervention needs. With Spradlin's permission, I modified this assessment tool (Sundberg, 1983) for use with younger children with language delays, and have since expanded on it in many ways (Partington & Sundberg, 1998; Sundberg, 2008, 2014; Sundberg & Partington, 1998). The *Verbal Behavior Milestones Assessment and Placement Program* (*VB-MAPP*) (Sundberg, 2014) is the most current version of an ABA/VB-based assessment tool. The VB-MAPP provides more information about an individual child than commonly used standardized language assessments (Esch et al., 2010). The VB-MAPP contains an assessment of 170 milestones across 16 language, play, and social domains that are developmentally matched to typical children. In addition, this tool contains an assessment of 24 language, learning, and social barriers that may impede progress and prevent a child from learning new skills. The VB-MAPP also contains a transition assessment to help determine what educational format might be of most value to a child (e.g., 1:1 instruction and/or group instruction, a center-based or inclusion program, DTT and/or NET) and help parents and educators make decisions. A list of supporting skills is also provided with an additional 700 skills that can be incorporated into an intervention program when appropriate. The final component of the VB-MAPP is a placement program that can be used to interpret the assessment results and guide an individualized educational program for a child.

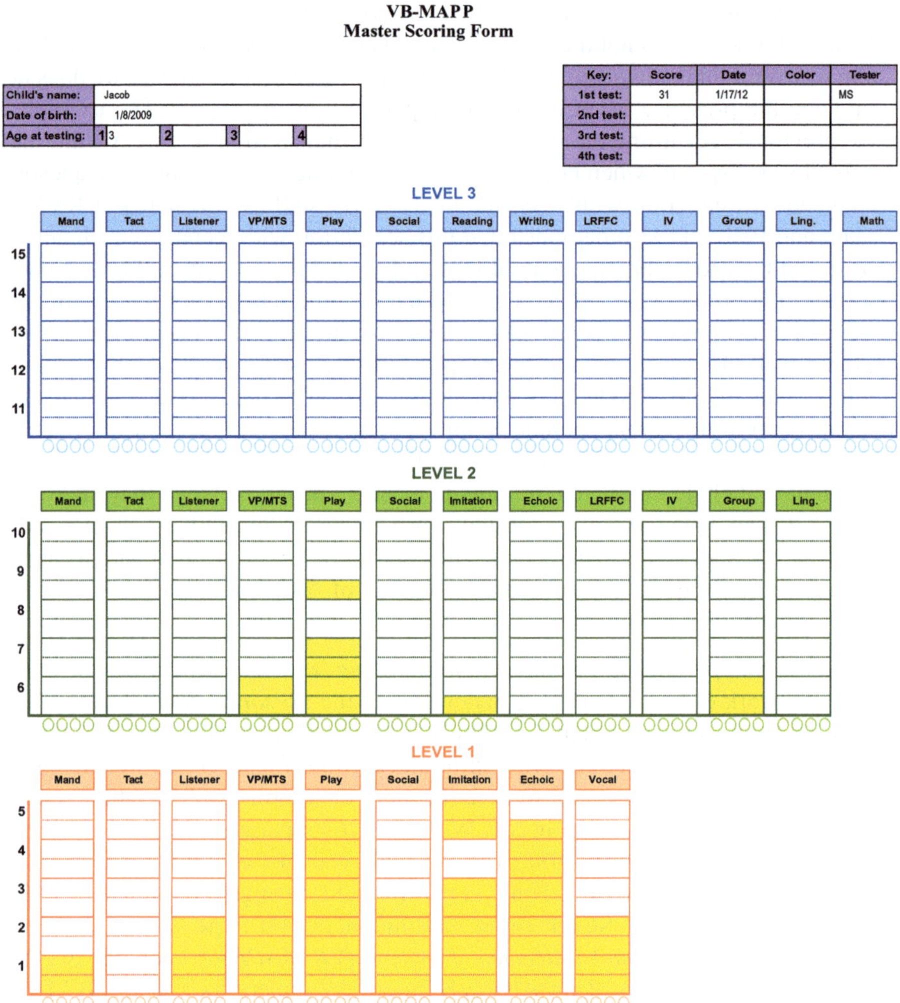

Fig. 5.1 An example of a 3-year-old child's VB-MAPP profile

A sample of a VB-MAPP Milestones assessment scoring form is presented in Fig. 5.1. This is the scoring form for Jacob, a 3-year-old boy with autism who does not emit any functional speech. His overall score on the VB-MAPP Milestones Assessment is in the Level 1 range as indicated by a score of 31 out of a possible score of 170. This places his language abilities around the developmental age of approximately 12–16 months. His comparative scores across domains are out of balance, demonstrating that some skills are much stronger than others. His general strengths are in the areas of visual perceptual and matching-to-sample skills, motor imitation, echoic, and play skills, while his weaknesses are in the areas of mand, tact, listener skills, and social skills (which constitute the primary domains of early language development and social behaviors). Jacob's VB-MAPP shows that a number of language and social skills are needed, and these should be the focus of his IEP and addressed in his daily intervention program. For example, his profile would suggest an intensive intervention program be implemented with the priorities being to establish a functional mand repertoire, free from echoic prompts, as well as targeting tacts, listener skills, social skills, and generalization of those skills. His strengths in the matching-to-sample, motor imitation, and echoic domains can be used to help teach mands, tacts, listener discriminations, and social skills (Sundberg, 2014).

Use the verbal operants as a framework for language intervention. A language intervention program for a child with autism should include training on all the verbal operants if needed, as well as on listener skills. Developmental norms should be considered and respected to help judge the appropriateness of the curriculum. The VB-MAPP can be used to guide that intervention program, insuring that each verbal operant is developed in a systematic manner. For example, if a child can emit listener discriminations, but not tacts, tact training should become an important part of his intervention program. Or, if he can tact, but not mand, then mand training should be included in the program. Ultimately, all of the verbal operants need to be developed and be reasonably balanced with each other. The VB-MAPP Barriers Assessment can help to identify specific problems a child may face, and lead to an individualized intervention program for those problems. For example, if a child is prompt-dependent, then specific procedures should be implemented to teach the child to self-initiate and be less dependent on prompts. But also, those implementing programming in the future should be careful to free responses from prompts during training. The book *Teaching language to children with autism or other developmental disabilities* (Sundberg & Partington, 1998) provides a verbal behavior-based intervention program that describes the basic training procedures for each of the verbal operants, as well as listener and matching skills.

Automatic reinforcement. Earlier, Bill Ahearn brought up the concept of automatic reinforcement in relation to problem behavior. This concept also plays a role in language acquisition. Skinner used the term automatic reinforcement in a number of his writings simply to indicate that reinforcement for a behavior can occur without someone directly providing it (Palmer, 1996; Vaughan & Michael, 1982). Automatic reinforcement, in lay terms, can occur because a behavior is fun to do (e.g., drawing, singing, self-stimulation) or has practical environment effects that are reinforcing (e.g., pushing on a door opens the door). There are many applications of this concept to skill acquisition for children with autism (Sundberg et al., 1996). For example, initially a child may need to be taught to imitate others, but eventually the child may imitate others because the behavior itself is fun and automatically reinforcing. This effect becomes obvious when the child independently emits adult behaviors (e.g., a funny walk, pretending to talk on a phone). It can be fun to act like mom or dad, sound like a movie or TV character, or follow peers who are running around. Again, the use of procedures to bring behavior under the control of automatic reinforcers is additive to existing ABA procedures (for a review of the research see Stock, Schulze, & Mirenda, 2008).

Multiple causation. One of the advantages of Skinner's functional analysis of language is that by clearly identifying the primary antecedent variable for each verbal operant, it is easy to identify situations where more than one variable is involved in evoking a specific response. Skinner calls this "multiple causation" (p. 227) and points out that most of our verbal behavior involves multiple antecedents and responses. Multiple causation pays an important role in our day-to-day behavior and constitutes a powerful analytical tool for understanding human behavior, especially verbal behavior (Michael et al., 2011). Incorporating this concept into assessment and intervention programs for children with language delays can have a significant impact on the correct development of some language skills. For example, if a child is asked "What color is that ball?" Saying "red" is multiply controlled by both the spoken word "color" and the actual color of the ball. If the question was "What shape is that ball?" A different word should be evoked, even though it is the same ball. The specific word emitted would depend on both the spoken word "shape" and the shape observed. This makes the response part tact and part intraverbal, and both sources of control are required to be correct. If a child emits a color word when asked a shape question, that would reveal that the relevant sources of multiple control were not affecting the child, thus suggesting the need for specific training.

Emerging (untrained) relations. An important aspect of language acquisition is often referred to as generative grammar, that is, new verbal responses occur without direct training (e.g., Alessi, 1987). For example, as a child learns to put verbs and nouns together (e.g., "push swing"), new combinations with different nouns and verbs usually occur without any formal instruction (e.g., "push wagon"). Thus, new verbal skills are said to emerge from existing skills and occur given novel combinations of variables in a child's daily environment. Skinner (1957) devoted several sections in *Verbal Behavior* to the analysis of emerging behavior (e.g., see Chap. 10), which has multiple applications to language intervention programs. An important contribution to the development of this area comes from the work of Sidman (1994) on equivalence relations, Horne and Lowe (1996) on naming, and Lowenkron (1998) on joint control. These three lines of research have produced extensive advancements in our understanding of emerging behavior and language acquisition (e.g., Causin, Albert, Carbone, & Sweeney-Kerwin, 2013; DeGraaf & Schlinger, 2012; Eikeseth & Smith, 1992; Horne, Lowe, & Randle, 2004; Kobari-Wright & Miguel, 2014; Lowenkron, 2006; Miguel, Petursdottir, Carr, & Michael, 2008; O'Donnell & Saunders, 2003; Perez-Gonzalez, Cereijo-Blanco, & Carnerero, 2014; Sidman & Tailby, 1982).

A Behavioral Analysis of Human Development

The third foundational aspect of the ABA/VB approach is a behavioral analysis of how a child learns and how human behavior becomes more complex. I refer here back to the work of Bijou and Baer. In the 1960s, they published a three-book *Child Development Series* (Bijou & Baer, 1961, 1965, 1967). These books contained the foundational aspects of a behavioral analysis of how children learn and develop throughout their early childhood. Their work has lead to a robust line of research and applications, as well as a dedicated journal (*Behavioral Development Bulletin*) and numerous extensions (e.g., Greer & Koehane, 2005; Morris et al., 1982; Novak & Pelaez, 2004; Schlinger, 1995). The VB-MAPP makes use of this aspect of behavior analysis in a number of ways, such as the developmental nature of the sequence of skills assessed, and comparisons of the acquisition of those skills to typical development (e.g., Sundberg & Sundberg, 2011). In addition, an ABA/VB intervention program makes use of Bijou and Baer's analysis of child learning when developing individualized intervention programs for children with autism.

A Behavioral Analysis of Language, Learning, and Social Barriers

The fourth component of an ABA/VB approach is the analysis and amelioration of barriers that can impede a child's language, learning, and social development. Several of these barriers address the second aspect of the DSM-5 criteria for the autism diagnosis "restricted and repetitive patterns of behavior" such as stereotypic or repetitive motor movements, inflexible adherence to routines, restricted or fixated interests, and sensory issues. These barriers may be quite complex and their treatment can be an ongoing aspect of a child's intervention program (e.g., behavior problems). In the VB-MAPP, I identify 24 barriers across six general categories (Sundberg, 2014). First, many children with autism or other intellectual disabilities exhibit strong and persistent negative behaviors that impede the teaching and learning process and make social interactions difficult (e.g., tantrums, aggression, self-injurious behaviors). Second, any one or more of the verbal operants or related skills may be absent, weak, or in some way impaired (e.g., echolalia, rote intraverbals). Third, social behavior can also become impaired for a variety of reasons (e.g., limited motivation for social interaction, or impaired mands). Fourth, there are several fundamental barriers to learning that must be analyzed and ameliorated to achieve significant gains (e.g., the failure to generalize, weak motivators, or prompt dependency). Fifth, there are a variety of specific behaviors that can compete with learning and social behavior (e.g., self-stimulation, hyperactive behavior, or sensory defensiveness). And, finally, some problems may be related to physical or medical barriers that must be accommodated or accounted for (e.g., sleep disorders, seizures, illnesses, allergies, cerebral palsy, visual and/or hearing impairments).

An intervention program for a child with autism should include both skills that need to be increased (e.g., mands, tacts, play, social skills, academics) and address behaviors or barriers that need to be decreased (e.g., tantrums, rote responding, sensory defensiveness). Often, it is the case that the absence of skills and the presence of barriers are closely related, and a comparison of a child's scores on both the Milestones Assessment and the Barriers Assessment can provide direction for a more focused intervention program. For example, the VB-MAPP Milestones

Assessment may show that a child needs to learn to mand (see Fig. 5.1), and this skill should be targeted for intervention with a focus on increasing the number of different mands that the child emits. However, the barriers assessment might reveal that a child is prompt-bound and scrolls (i.e., guesses) through words. These two barriers would need to be removed in order for the mand repertoire to grow and become functional for the child. Thus, the intervention program should contain a careful focus on freeing the child's mands from prompts and eliminate scrolling when manding. New barriers or recurring barriers can emerge at any point and can only be ameliorated if and when detected.

Conceptual Basis for the ABA/VB Approach

The conceptual foundation of the ABA/VB approach is from the field of behavior analysis in general (Skinner, 1953) and the analysis of verbal behavior in particular (Skinner, 1957). As previously mentioned, the concepts and principles of behavior analysis provide the basic foundations for this approach and drive the intervention. I would like to provide an example of how the four foundational aspects of the ABA/VB approach can be used to better understand and treat the language training needs faced by children with autism.

ABA/VB Foundation 1: The concepts and principles of behavior analysis. Consider the problem of a child with autism's inability to ask questions. What principles of behavior are involved in asking questions? What is the relevant antecedent source of control for a child asking, for example, "When is mommy coming home?" Would it be an MO or an S^D? These are two separate sources of control. The answer is that questions should be under the functional control of MOs, specifically MOs for verbal information (Skinner, 1957). That is, when the value of information regarding when mother is coming home is strong, it should evoke a specific behavior (a verbal question). The reinforcement for this behavior is specific to the MO for information (providing the time of arrival). If a child is not able to ask questions, or his question-asking repertoire is impaired in some way, then intervention procedures such as modeling, prompting, fading, and differential reinforcement can be used to teach the skill. Data are collected and learning can be measured. If learning is not occurring, adjustments to the intervention program should be made.

ABA/VB Foundation 2: Skinner's (1957) analysis of verbal behavior. How does Skinner's analysis of language help us with the analysis of question asking? Asking questions would be classified as mands given the causal role of the MO and specific reinforcement. These mands for information are not the same as echoics, tacts, or intraverbals. This analysis would drive the intervention program with the goal of being assured that the target response is primarily controlled by an MO, not a verbal or nonverbal S^D. Thus, the intervention procedure would require that an MO for information be captured or created, followed by the implementation of ABA techniques (e.g., prompting, reinforcement) to bring the verbal response under the control of the relevant MO (e.g., Lechago, Carr, Grow, Love, & Almason, 2010; Shillingsburg & Valentino, 2010; Sundberg, Loeb, Hale, & Eigenheer, 2002).

ABA/VB Foundation 3: A behavioral analysis of human development. What does an analysis of typical human development and language acquisition tell us? Mands for information are relatively late in language development. That is, functionally correct WH questions may not begin to appear in the verbal repertoire of typically developing children until around the age of two (Brown et al., 1969). But by 2 years of age, a typically developing child has anywhere from 100 to 200 mands and tacts, with noun–verb combinations, and a high rate of daily verbal output, and they are just beginning to ask functionally correct WH questions. If a child with autism does not demonstrate this level of prerequisite verbal behavior, an intervention program for asking questions may not be appropriate at this time.

ABA/VB Foundation 4: A behavioral analysis of potential barriers. It also may be possible that a focus on WH questions too soon could produce rote question asking that becomes difficult to ameliorate (e.g., an MO for information may not be the source of control for the question-asking behavior). A child might learn to ask questions that appear structurally correct, but are not functionally correct. For example, a child with autism might learn to walk up to somebody and say, "What's your name?," but walks away before the peer says his name. He may look to a staff member who may give him an edible or token for initiating the verbal interaction with the peer, but this behavior is not under the control of an MO for information, or the reinforcement relevant to that MO, rather it is controlled by S^Ds, tokens, and praise, and not a functionally correct question.

Primary Procedural Components

I will now provide a brief overview of the main components of the ABA/VB teaching methodology. The first element of an ABA/VB program is an assessment of a child's verbal and nonverbal skills, as well as his barriers to learning, with a tool such as the VB-MAPP. Once a profile is obtained, priorities can be determined, IEP goals set, and an intervention program designed. Like all ABA approaches, an intensive style of intervention constitutes the educational format offered to the child. By intensive, I mean several hours a day of direct teaching of the skills that a child may need, with a high rate of active responding on the part of the child. Instruction is conducted in multiple daily structured teaching sessions (DTT), as well as teaching in the child's natural environment (NET). The teaching procedures used are those derived from the field of applied behavior analysis (e.g., Cooper et al., 2007) and are common to most ABA style programs (prompting, fading, shaping, reinforcing). Data are collected daily with an emphasis on a "first trial correct" mastery criteria measurement system. For example, given a particular target, on the first trial of the day, (e.g., a tact for wheel), the first response emitted by the child must be correct for 3 days in a row. Once a word is acquired in this manner, it is then moved to generalization, integration with the other domains, and expansion that involves various combinations with other parts of speech (e.g., noun–verb combinations).

As previously mentioned, the most unique aspect of the ABA/VB approach is the use of Skinner's analysis of verbal behavior as the foundation for the assessment and intervention program. With typical language development serving as a curriculum guide, the goal is to establish each verbal operant for a child, beginning with developmentally appropriate, fun, and engaging skills and systematically progressing to more complex skills. Every effort should be made to make teaching and learning reinforcing and functional for the child. The child's daily schedule and IEP goals are primarily focused on developing the verbal operants, social behavior, academic behavior, as well as other related skills. Given the role of the mand in language development, and its early appearance in the repertoires of most typically developing children, establishing a functional mand repertoire is an early and ongoing instructional target for many children with autism. Continuing efforts are made to integrate each verbal operant with the other verbal and listener domains (mands, tacts, intraverbals, listener discriminations), and with nonverbal behavior, social behavior, academic behavior, activities of daily living, and so on. In order to facilitate this, and novel responding, creativity, and generative linguistic behavior, a "mixed verbal behavior" teaching format with multiple exemplars is often (but not exclusively) used. With this format, multiple exemplars of the verbal operants are interspersed with each other, including examples and non-examples, in a given teaching session (e.g., a tact trial, then a listener trial, then a mand trial). This same teaching strategy is also used for instruction in the child's natural environment.

There is also an emphasis on a child's ongoing MOs and reinforcing and expanding child-initiated behaviors (e.g., Hart & Risley, 1975). Opportunities to mand are frequent and often used as a form of reinforcement for other correct verbal and nonverbal behaviors. Augmentative and Alternative communication (AAC) is used when necessary for individual children, but there is always a primary focus on speech if possible. Sign language is generally the preferred type of AAC for a variety of reasons (Sundberg, 1993; Sundberg & Sundberg, 1990), but icon selection or textual stimuli can be effective when appropriate. There is also a strong focus on teaching verbal and social interaction with peers and developing both social and independent play skills. More advanced language skills (e.g., intraverbals, adjectives, pronouns) are taught by building on known skills (e.g., tacts, nouns, verbs) and are systematically incorporated into all the verbal operants guided by developmental norms. There is a strong focus on parent training and their involvement in the intervention program.

How Goals Are Selected and Sequenced

The VB-MAPP (Sundberg, 2014) can be used to establish a child's baseline skills across 16 domains, 24 barriers, and 18 transition areas. As previously mentioned, the VB-MAPP contains a developmentally based sequence of language and social skills that can be used to guide the content of the treatment program. The data from this assessment are used to identify priorities and establish IEP goals for a child. For example, the VB-MAPP profile I presented for Jacob previously indicates that he needs an intensive intervention program with the immediate priorities being to establish a mand repertoire, free from echoic prompts, as well as targeting tacts, listener skills, and social skills. A barriers assessment would also be used to identify any specific problems that might warrant IEP goals (e.g., non compliance, aggression). Others such as SLPs, occupational therapists, and parents might add additional targets. The placement section of the VB-MAPP provides direction in selecting specific goals for a child. Each domain contains a list of sample IEP goals, with over 200 goals provided in total. These suggested goals can be adjusted to meet the needs of an individual child. The VB-MAPP is developmentally sequenced in an effort to target skills that match those of typically developing children at the various performance levels. For example, if a child can tact at least 100 individual nouns and verbs, work should begin on developing noun–verb two word combinations both as a speaker and as a listener, which is a well-accepted 2-year linguistic milestone for typically developing children.

Staff Skills and Required Training

The problems faced by a child with autism are complex and widely varied and usually require a highly specialized intervention program to achieve meaningful gains. Behavioral approaches have been demonstrated to be the most effective (National Standards Project, 2014), but they require an extensive skill set on the part of those conducting the intervention. First, supervisors and hands-on staff must be proficient in a large number of different ABA procedures and data collection methods (e.g., Cooper et al., 2007), any of which could play a role in a given child's program (e.g., shaping, prompting, chaining, tokens, probe measures). A program for children with autism should include a structured staff training component that contains both the academic content of behavior analysis and hands-on supervision, training, and monitoring from those who are already proficient in behavioral concepts (e.g., a BCBA). This process can take several years, and can be on-going, but without it an intervention program is likely to be less successful.

The second significant skill set required to implement an ABA/VB program is a working knowledge of the basic concepts and the procedures derived from Skinner's analysis of verbal behavior (e.g., MO manipulation, mand training, intraverbal training). Given that social communication deficits constitute the major diagnostic criteria for autism, an intervention program without a focus on language cannot possibly address a child's needs. The question is what theory of language, of the many choices, will provide the best conceptual foundation necessary to guide a language intervention program? It is suggested here that Skinner's behavioral formulation provides the most value for children with autism. In addition to procedures relevant to ABA and Skinner's analysis verbal behavior, staff must also learn the basic aspects of structural linguistics, and how to integrate these systems. For example, there are different procedures for teaching adjectives and prepositions as tacts versus teaching adjectives and prepositions as intraverbals.

There are a variety of additional skills that are necessary for working with children with autism. Supervisors should be in touch with the body of research on autism that is available in the literature. Knowledge in the area of child development is also quite important to understanding what typical children at various ages are capable of doing, along with the analysis of how they learn the skills they have. Such an analysis can provide both a curriculum guide as well as comparison data regarding a child's progress. In addition, specific experience with autism or other intellectual disabilities may be useful for staff to have. This experience could be acquired in formal college coursework, as well as hands-on supervised training. Given the wide range of issues children with autism often present, the more varied a person's contact is with this population, the more prepared he or she will be when facing new children and new challenges.

Finally, it is important that parents of children with autism receive as much of the same basic training as possible; realizing, of course, that may be difficult for some families and resources may be limited. However, parents who do acquire basic ABA/VB skills are in a much better position to work with their children and provide teaching moments throughout the child's day. Some possible ways to provide support for parents include: (1) provide a weekly or monthly parent training class, (2) provide weekly small group parent discussions moderated by the BCBA, SLP, or classroom teacher, (3) provide in-classroom demonstrations of the procedures for the parents to observe, (4) have the parents practice those procedures and provide them with feedback, (5) give the parents homework assignments, (6) teach parents how to read and collect data, (7) teach parents how to interpret and use the VB-MAPP, (8) provide the parents with user-friendly material on ABA and verbal behavior (e.g., Barbera & Rasmussen, 2007; Reynolds, 2013; Schramm, 2011; Sundberg & Partington, 1998; Weiss & Demiri, 2011), and (9) provide parents with links to internet information that will help them, rather than confuse them.

The Evidence Base

The foundation of ABA/VB comes directly from the well-established field of behavior analysis. It makes specific use of the scientific principles of human behavior (Skinner, 1953) to guide assessment and intervention procedures used for children with language delays. Its origins can be traced back to the founders of our field and the initial application of behavioral principles to autism treatment. The systematic inclusion of Skinner's analysis of verbal behavior is a novel contribution compared to other ABA approaches, but that too is based on a solid foundation of empirical behavioral data. There is now an extensive body of outcome studies showing the positive effects of ABA methodology (e.g., Eikeseth, Smith, Jahr, & Eldevik, 2002; Howard, Sparkman, Cohen, Green, & Stanislaw, 2005; Lovaas, 1987). Some

ABA intervention outcome studies have included aspects of a verbal behavior program such as a mand training component (e.g., Sallows & Graupner, 2005), and there are many studies demonstrating the effectiveness of the individual components of an ABA/VB program (e.g., Sautter & LeBlanc, 2006).

Perhaps the most immediate contribution of Skinner's analysis of verbal behavior to ABA and work with children with autism may be that it provides an organized and thorough way to analyze language. With ASD being characterized by communication challenges and social interaction difficulties, a verbal behavior analysis can be used to identify and quantify language deficits and provide direction and guidance for language intervention programs. There are many thematic lines of empirical research emanating directly from Skinner's analysis of verbal behavior that have directly benefited children with autism. For example, research on the distinction between the verbal operants has demonstrated that mands may not emerge from tact training (e.g., Gamba, Goyos, & Petursdottir, 2015; Hall & Sundberg, 1987; Shafer, 1994; Twyman, 1996). Also, there are data to support that intraverbal behavior may not emerge from tact training (e.g., Braam & Poling, 1983; Goldsmith, LeBlanc, & Sautter, 2007; Ingvarsson & Duy, 2011; Luciano, 1986). On the other hand, there are circumstances where these operants are interdependent and transfer among them and listener discriminations occur with little or no formal training (Gamba et al., 2015; Horne & Lowe, 1996; Miguel et al., 2008; Wallace, Iwata, & Hanley, 2006). Collectively, this extensive line of research provides empirical support for the importance of distinguishing between the verbal operants for children with autism. At the least, an intervention program that respects these distinctions seems to be an improvement over those that neglect them.

There are a number of empirical studies on teaching language to children with autism that are based on Skinner's analysis of verbal behavior. For example, two different thematic lines of research on mand training provide support for Skinner's conceptual analysis of that verbal operant. First, the extensive work on functional communication training initiated by Carr and Durand (1985) demonstrates how an alternative and acceptable mand form can replace a mand form consisting of aggressive or self-injurious behavior. Second, the research mentioned previously on manding for information has provided immediate applications to autism treatment (e.g., Endicott & Higbee, 2007; Lechago et al., 2010; Shillingsburg & Valentino, 2010; Sundberg et al., 2002). Another body of research addresses Skinner's analysis of the distinction between the behavior of the speaker and behavior of the listener, and data show, like Skinner suggested, they are functionally independent repertoires (e.g., Lee, 1981). However, the speaker and listener repertoires can interact in a number of important ways as described by Skinner (1957), such as the "naming" repertoire identified by Horne and Lowe (1996). The naming literature is now quite extensive and has significant implications for the emergence of untrained types of verbal behavior from those that have been formally trained (e.g., Eikeseth & Smith, 1992; Horne, Hughes, & Lowe, 2006; Kobari-Wright & Miguel, 2014; Lowe, Horne, & Hughes, 2005; Miguel et al., 2008; Perez-Gonzalez et al., 2014; Randell & Remington, 1999). Lowenkron's (1984, 1988, 1989, 1998, 2006) work on joint control also addresses the issue of emergence of untrained behaviors with a strong collection of data demonstrating the effects of combining the verbal operants (multiple control) in generating new behavioral relations (Michael et al., 2011). Valuable applications based on this line of research are also available in the literature (e.g., Causin, Albert, Carbone, & Sweeney-Kerwin, 2013).

Greer and colleagues (e.g., Greer & Ross, 2007) have published an extensive collection of verbal behavior research projects over the past 30 years that have produced a number of important findings, such as the value of multiple exemplar training in establishing the verbal operants (e.g., Greer, Yuan, & Gautreaux, 2005). A growing body of empirical research also exists on Skinner's analysis of automatic reinforcement and its relation to language acquisition, as well as autism treatment (Smith, Michael, & Sundberg, 1996; Stock et al., 2008; Sundberg et al., 1996; Yoon & Bennett, 2000). Michael's (1985) distinction between topography-based verbal behavior and selection-based verbal behavior has generated a number of research projects that have provided conceptual and empirical clarity to the issue of using sign language versus icon selection-based communication systems for children with autism (Lowenkron, 1991; Shafer, 1993; Sundberg & Sundberg, 1990; Wraikat, Sundberg, & Michael, 1991). Hundreds of additional studies on a wide range of verbal behavior topics can be found in various journals (e.g., TAVB, JABA, JEAB, JEIBI, ETC). In fact, it is now quite common to see empirical studies based on verbal behavior in most issues of JABA. Several reviews of various aspects of verbal behavior research and practices are also available in the literature (e.g., Carr & Petursdottir, 2011; Gamba et al., 2015; Oah & Dickinson, 1989; Sautter & LeBlanc, 2006; Shafer, 1994; Stock et al., 2008), as well as reviews of the publication trends in the journal, *The Analysis of Verbal Behavior* (Luke & Carr, 2015; Petursdottir, Peterson, & Peters, 2009). The data seem to indicate that there no longer appears to be a shortage of verbal behavior research (Carr & Firth, 2005; Sundberg, 1991).

Conclusion

The primary focus of an intervention program for a child with autism should be on the development of effective language and social skills, as well as the reduction of negative behaviors. Behavior analysis has much to offer this effort. ABA is a scientifically based analysis of human behavior (Skinner, 1953) that has generated a robust applied field that produces a steady stream of applications for ameliorating various human problems (e.g., Cooper et al., 2007) and has undoubtedly benefitted many children with ASD. Skinner's (1957) analysis of verbal behavior adds to existing ABA programs by providing a behavioral analysis of language that is also based on a foundation of empirical research. The benefits of Skinner's analysis of verbal behavior are substantial and provide for greater consistency between the conceptual and applied aspects of an intervention program (Hedge, 2010). A behavior analysis of child development can contribute further to an intervention program by providing a framework for sequencing language and other skills. Finally, the analysis and amelioration of language, learning, and social barriers experienced by a child with autism is an essential component of an intervention program, but may require professionals with advanced skills in behavior analysis. Collectively, these foundational aspects of an ABA/VB program can provide specific evidenced-based guidance for the development of an intervention program for a child with autism.

References

Alessi, G. (1987). Generative strategies and teaching for generalization. *The Analysis of Verbal Behavior, 5*, 15–27.

Axe, J. B. (2008). Conditional discrimination in the intraverbal relation: A review and recommendations for future research. *The Analysis of Verbal Behavior, 24*, 159–174.

Ayllon, T., & Azrin, N. H. (1968). *The token economy: A motivational system for therapy and rehabilitation*. New York: Appleton.

Ayllon, T., & Michael, J. (1959). The psychiatric nurse as a behavioral engineer. *Journal of the Experimental Analysis of Behavior, 2*, 323–334.

Barbera, M. L., & Rasmussen, T. (2007). *The verbal behavior approach*. London: Jessica Kingsley.

Bijou, S. W., & Baer, D. M. (1961). *Child development I: A systematic and empirical theory*. Englewood Cliffs, NJ: Prentice-Hall.

Bijou, S. W., & Baer, D. M. (1965). *Child development II: Universal stage of infancy*. Englewood Cliffs, NJ: Prentice-Hall.

Bijou, S. W., & Baer, D. M. (1967). *Child development III: Readings in the experimental analysis*. Englewood Cliffs, NJ: Prentice-Hall.

Braam, S. J., & Poling, A. (1983). Development of intraverbal behavior in mentally retarded individuals through transfer of stimulus control procedures: Classification of verbal responses. *Applied Research in Mental Retardation, 4*, 279–302.

Brown, R. (1973). *A first language: The early stages*. Cambridge, MA: Harvard University Press.

Brown, R., Cazden, C., & Bellugi, U. (1969). The child's grammar from I to III. In J. P. Hill (Ed.), *The 1967 symposium on child psychology* (pp. 28–73). Minneapolis, MN: University of Minnesota Press.

Bruner, J. S. (1983). *Child's talk*. New York: Norton.

Carbone, V. J. (2013). The establishing operation and teaching verbal behavior. *The Analysis of Verbal Behavior, 29*, 45–49.

Carr, E. G., & Durand, V. M. (1985). Reducing behavior problems through functional communication training. *Journal of Applied Behavior Analysis, 18*, 111–126.

Carr, J. E., & Firth, A. M. (2005). The verbal behavior approach to early and intensive behavioral intervention for autism: A call for additional empirical support. *Journal of Early and Intensive Behavioral Intervention, 2*, 18–27.

Carr, J. E., & Petursdottir, A. I. (2011). A review of recommendations for sequencing receptive and expressive language instruction. *Journal of Applied Behavior Analysis, 44*, 859–876.

Causin, K. G., Albert, K. M., Carbone, V. J., & Sweeney-Kerwin, E. J. (2013). The role of joint control in teaching listener responding to children with autism and other developmental disabilities. *Research in Autism Spectrum Disorders, 7*, 997–1011.

Chomsky, N. (1957). *Syntactic structures*. The Hague: Mouton.

Chomsky, N. (1959). Review of B. F. Skinner's *verbal behavior. Language, 35*, 26–58.

Cooper, J. O., Heron, T. E., & Heward, W. L. (2007). *Applied behavior analysis* (2nd ed.). Upper Saddle River, NJ: Merrill/Prentice-Hall.

DeGraaf, A., & Schlinger, H. (2012). The effect of joint control training on the acquisition and durability of a sequencing task. *The Analysis of Verbal Behavior, 28*, 59–71.

Dunn, L. M., & Dunn, D. M. (2007). *Peabody picture vocabulary test* (4th ed.). San Antonio, TX: Pearson.

Eikeseth, S., & Smith, T. (1992). The development of functional and equivalence classes in high-functioning autistic children: The role of naming. *Journal of the Experimental Analysis of Behavior, 58*, 123–133.

Eikeseth, S., & Smith, D. P. (2013). An analysis of verbal stimulus control in intraverbal behavior: Implications for practice and applied research. *The Analysis of Verbal Behavior, 29*, 125–135.

Eikeseth, S., Smith, T., Jahr, E., & Eldevik, S. (2002). Intensive behavioral treatment at school for 4–7-year-old children with autism: A 1-year comparison controlled study. *Behavior Modification, 2002*, 49–68.

Endicott, K., & Higbee, T. S. (2007). Contriving motivating operations to evoke mands for information in preschoolers with autism. *Research in Autism Spectrum Disorders, 1*, 210–217.

Esch, B. E., LaLonde, K. B., & Esch, J. W. (2010). Speech and language assessment: A verbal behavior analysis. *The Journal of Speech-Language Pathology and Applied Behavior Analysis, 5*, 166–191.

Ferster, C. B. (1961). Positive reinforcement and behavioral deficits of autistic children. *Child Development, 32*, 437–456.

Ferster, C. B., & DeMyer, M. K. (1962). A method for the experimental analysis of the autistic child. *American Journal of Orthopsychiatry, 32*, 89–98.

Gamba, J., Goyos, C., & Petursdottir, A. I. (2015). The functional independence of mands and tacts: Has it been demonstrated empirically? *The Analysis of Verbal Behavior, 31*, 10–38.

Ghezzi, P. M. (2010). In memoriam: Sidney W. Bijou. *Journal of Applied Behavior Analysis, 43*, 175–179.

Goldsmith, T. R., LeBlanc, L. A., & Sautter, R. A. (2007). Teaching intraverbal behavior to children with autism. *Research in Autism Spectrum Disorders, 1*, 1–13.

Greer, R. D., & Koehane, D. (2005). The evolution of verbal behavior in children. *Behavioral Development, 1*, 31–48.

Greer, R. D., & Ross, D. E. (2007). *Verbal behavior analysis*. New York: Allyn & Bacon.

Greer, R. D., Yuan, L., & Gautreaux, G. (2005). Novel dictation and intraverbal responses as a function of a multiple exemplar history. *The Analysis of Verbal Behavior, 21*, 99–116.

Hall, G. A., & Sundberg, M. L. (1987). Teaching mands by manipulating conditioned establishing operations. *The Analysis of Verbal Behavior, 5*, 41–53.

Hart, B., & Risley, T. R. (1975). Incidental teaching of language in the preschool. *Journal of Applied Behavior Analysis, 8*, 411–420.

Hedge, H. M. (2010). Language and grammar: A behavioral analysis. *The Journal of Speech-Language Pathology and Applied Behavior Analysis, 5*, 90–113.

Horne, P. J., Hughes, J. C., & Lowe, C. F. (2006). Naming and categorization in young children: IV: Listener behavior training and transfer of function. *Journal of the Experimental Analysis of Behavior, 85*, 247–273.

Horne, P. J., & Lowe, C. F. (1996). On the origins of naming and other symbolic behavior. *Journal of the Experimental Analysis of Behavior, 65*, 185–241.

Horne, P. J., Lowe, C. F., & Randle, V. R. L. (2004). Naming and categorization in young children: II. Listener behavior training. *Journal of the Experimental Analysis of Behavior, 81*, 267–288.

Howard, J. S., Sparkman, C. R., Cohen, H. G., Green, G., & Stanislaw, H. (2005). A comparison of intensive behavior analytic and eclectic treatments for young children with autism. *Research in Developmental Disabilities, 26*, 359–383.

Ingvarsson, E. T., & Duy, D. L. (2011). Further evaluation of prompting tactics for establishing intraverbal responding in children with autism. *The Analysis of Verbal Behavior, 27*, 75–93.

Kobari-Wright, V. V., & Miguel, C. F. (2014). The effects of listener training on the emergence of categorization and speaker behavior in children with autism. *Journal of Applied Behavior Analysis, 47*, 1–6.

Koegel, R. L., O'Dell, M. C., & Koegel, L. K. (1987). A natural language paradigm for teaching autistic children. *Journal of Autism and Developmental Disabilities, 17*, 187–199.

Lechago, S. A., Carr, J. E., Grow, L. L., Love, J. R., & Almason, S. M. (2010). Mands for information generalize across establishing operations. *Journal of Applied Behavior Analysis, 43*, 381–395.
Lee, V. L. (1981). Prepositional phrases spoken and heard. *Journal of the Experimental Analysis of Behavior, 35*, 227–242.
Lovaas, O. I. (1977). *The autistic child: Language development through behavior modification*. New York: Irvington.
Lovaas, O. I. (1987). Behavioral treatment and normal educational and intellectual functioning in young autistic children. *Journal of Consulting and Clinical Psychology, 55*, 3–9.
Lovaas, O. I. (2003). *Teaching individuals with developmental delays*. Austin TX: Pro-ed.
Lowe, C. F., Horne, P. J., & Hughes, J. C. (2005). Naming and categorization in young children: III. Vocal tact training and transfer of function. *Journal of the Experimental Analysis of Behavior, 83*, 47–65.
Lowenkron, B. (1984). Coding responses and the generalization of matching to sample in children. *Journal of the Experimental Analysis of Behavior, 42*, 1–18.
Lowenkron, B. (1988). Generalization of delayed identity matching in retarded children. *Journal of the Experimental Analysis of Behavior, 50*, 163–172.
Lowenkron, B. (1989). Instructional control of generalized relational matching to sample in children. *Journal of the Experimental Analysis of Behavior, 52*, 293–309.
Lowenkron, B. (1991). Joint control and the generalization of selection-based verbal behavior. *The Analysis of Verbal Behavior, 9*, 121–126.
Lowenkron, B. (1998). Some logical functions of joint control. *Journal of the Experimental Analysis of Behavior, 69*, 327–354.
Lowenkron, B. (2006). Joint control and the selection of stimuli from their description. *The Analysis of Verbal Behavior, 22*, 129–151.
Luciano, C. (1986). Acquisition, maintenance, and generalization of productive intraverbal behavior through transfer of stimulus control procedures. *Applied Research in Mental Retardation, 7*, 1–20.
Luke, M. M., & Carr, J. E. (2015). The analysis of verbal behavior: A status update. *The Analysis of Verbal Behavior, 31*, 153–161.
Malott, R. W., & Shane, J. T. (2013). *Principles of behavior* (7th ed.). New York: Routledge.
Martin, G. L., & Pear, J. J. (2015). *Behavior modification: What is it and how to do it* (10th ed.). New York: Routledge.
Maurice, C., Green, G., & Luce, S. C. (1996). *Behavior interventions for young children with autism*. Austin, TX: Pro-ed.
McGreevy, P., Fry, T., & Cornwall, C. (2012). *Essentials for living*. Winter Park, FL: Patrick McGreevy.
McNeill, D. (1970). *The acquisition of language*. New York: Harper and Row.
Meyerson, L., & Michael, J. (1964). Assessment of hearing by operant conditioning. In *Report of the proceedings of the international congress on education of the deaf* (pp. 237–242). Washington: U.S. Government Printing Office.
Michael, J. (1982). Skinner's elementary verbal relations: Some new categories. *The Analysis of Verbal Behavior, 1*, 1–4.
Michael, J. (1984). Verbal behavior. *Journal of the Experimental Analysis of Behavior, 42*, 363–376.
Michael, J. (1985). Two kinds of verbal behavior plus a possible third. *The Analysis of Verbal Behavior, 3*, 1–4.
Michael, J. (1988). Establishing operations and the mand. *The Analysis of Verbal Behavior, 6*, 3–9.
Michael, J. (2004). *Concepts and principles of behavior analysis* (2nd ed.). Kalamazoo, MI: Association for Behavior Analysis International.
Michael, J. (2007). Motivating operations. In J. O. Cooper, T. E. Heron, & W. L. Heward (Eds.), *Applied behavior analysis* (2nd ed., pp. 374–391). Upper Saddle River, NJ: Merrill/Prentice Hall.

Michael, J., Palmer, D. C., & Sundberg, M. L. (2011). The multiple control of verbal behavior. *The Analysis of Verbal Behavior, 27*, 3–22.
Miguel, C. F., Petursdottir, A. I., Carr, J. E., & Michael, J. (2008). The role of naming in stimulus categorization by preschool children. *Journal of the Experimental Analysis of Behavior, 89*, 383–405.
Miltenberger, R. G. (2015). *Behavior modification: Principles and procedures* (6th ed.). Pacific Grove, CA: Cengage/Wadsworth.
Morris, E. K., Hursh, D. E., Winston, A. S., Gelfand, D. M., Hartmann, D. P., Reese, H. W., & Baer, D. M. (1982). Behavior analysis and developmental psychology. *Human Development,* 25, 340–364.
Morris, E. K., Smith, N. G., & Altus, D. E. (2005). B. F. Skinner's contributions to applied behavior analysis. *The Behavior Analyst, 28*, 99–131.
National Standards Project. (2014). Randolph, MA: National Autism Center.
Normand, M. P. (2009). Much ado about nothing? Some comments on B. F. Skinner's definition of verbal behavior. *The Behavior Analyst, 32*, 185–190.
Novak, G., & Pelaez, M. (2004). *Child and adolescent development: A behavioral systems approach*. Thousand Oaks, CA: Sage.
O'Donnell, J., & Saunders, K. J. (2003). Equivalence relations in individuals with language limitations and mental retardation. *Journal of the Experimental Analysis of Behavior, 80*, 131–157.
Oah, S., & Dickinson, A. M. (1989). A review of empirical studies of verbal behavior. *The Analysis of Verbal Behavior, 7*, 53–68.
Palmer, D. C. (1996). Achieving parity: The role of automatic reinforcement. *Journal of the Experimental Analysis of Behavior, 65*, 289–290.
Partington, J. W., & Sundberg, M. L. (1998). *The assessment of basic language and learning skills (The ABLLS)*. Pleasant Hill, CA: Behavior Analysts.
Perez-Gonzalez, L. A., Cereijo-Blanco, N., & Carnerero, J. J. (2014). Emerging tacts and selections from previous learned skills: A comparison between two types of naming. *The Analysis of Verbal Behavior, 30*, 184–192.
Petursdottir, A. I., Peterson, S. P., & Peters, A. C. (2009). A quarter century of the analysis of verbal behavior: An analysis of impact. *The Analysis of Verbal Behavior, 25*, 109–121.
Piaget, J. (1952). *The origins of intelligence in children* (M. Cook, Trans.). New York: International University Press.
Pinker, S. (1994). *The language instinct: How the mind creates language*. New York: Harper-Collins.
Randell, T., & Remington, B. (1999). Equivalence relations between visual stimuli: The functional role of naming. *Journal of the Experimental Analysis of Behavior, 71*, 395–415.
Reynolds, R. (2013). *Teaching children with autism: An ABA primer*. Lulu Enterprises.
Sallows, G. O., & Graupner, T. D. (2005). Intensive behavioral treatment for children with autism: Four-year outcome and predictors. *American Journal on Mental Retardation, 110*, 417–438.
Saunders, K. J., & Spradlin, J. E. (1989). Conditional discrimination in mentally retarded adults: The effect of training the component simple discriminations. *Journal of the Experimental Analysis of Behavior, 52*, 1–12.
Sautter, R. A., & LeBlanc, L. A. (2006). Empirical applications of Skinner's analysis of verbal behavior with humans. *The Analysis of Verbal Behavior, 22*, 35–48.
Schlinger, H. D., Jr. (1995). *A behavior analytic view of child development*. New York: Springer.
Schlinger, H. D., Jr. (2008). Listening is behaving verbally. *The Behavior Analyst, 31*, 145–161.
Schramm, R. (2011). *Motivation and reinforcement: Turning the tables on autism*. Lulu Enterprises.
Shafer, E. (1993). Teaching topography-based and selection-based verbal behavior to developmentally disabled individuals: Some considerations. *The Analysis of Verbal Behavior, 11*, 117–133.
Shafer, E. (1994). A review of interventions to teach a mand repertoire. *The Analysis of Verbal Behavior, 12*, 53–66.

Shillingsburg, M. A., & Valentino, A. L. (2010). Teaching a child with autism to mand for information using "how". *The Analysis of Verbal Behavior, 27*, 179–184.

Sidman, M. (1994). *Equivalence relations and behavior: A research story*. Boston: Authors Cooperative.

Sidman, M., & Tailby, W. (1982). Conditional discrimination vs. matching to sample: An expansion of the testing paradigm. *Journal of the Experimental Analysis of Behavior, 37*, 23–44.

Skinner, B. F. (1953). *Science and human behavior*. New York: Free Press.

Skinner, B. F. (1957). *Verbal behavior*. New York: Appleton.

Slobin, D. I. (1973). Cognitive prerequisites for the development of grammar. In C. A. Ferguson & D. I. Slobin (Eds.), *Studies of child language development* (pp. 175–202). New York: Holt, Rinehart, and Winston.

Smith, R., Michael, J., & Sundberg, M. L. (1996). Automatic reinforcement and automatic punishment in infant vocal behavior. *The Analysis of Verbal Behavior, 13*, 39–48.

Spradlin, J. E. (1963). Assessment of speech and language of retarded children: The Parsons language sample. *Journal of Speech and Hearing Disorders Monograph, 10*, 8–31.

Spradlin, J. E. (1966). Environmental factors and the language development of retarded children. In S. Rosenberg (Ed.), *Developments in applied psycholinguist research* (pp. 261–290). Riverside, NJ: MacMillan.

Stafford, M. W., Sundberg, M. L., & Braam, S. J. (1988). A preliminary investigation of the consequences that define the mand and the tact. *The Analysis of Verbal Behavior, 6*, 61–71.

Stock, R. A., Schulze, K. A., & Mirenda, P. (2008). A comparison of stimulus-stimulus pairing, standard echoic training, and control procedures, of the vocal behavior of children with autism. *The Analysis of Verbal Behavior, 24*, 123–133.

Sulzer-Azaroff, B., Mayer, G. R., & Wallace, M. (2013). *Behavior analysis for lasting change*. Cornwell-on-Hudson, NY: Sloan.

Sundberg, C. T., & Sundberg, M. L. (1990). Comparing topography-based verbal behavior with stimulus selection-based verbal behavior. *The Analysis of Verbal Behavior, 8*, 31–41.

Sundberg, M. L. (1980). *Developing a verbal repertoire using sign language and Skinner's analysis of verbal behavior* (Unpublished doctoral dissertation, Western Michigan University).

Sundberg, M. L. (1983). Language. In J. L. Matson & S. E. Breuning (Eds.), *Assessing the mentally retarded* (pp. 285–310). New York: Grune & Stratton.

Sundberg, M. L. (1991). 301 research topics from Skinner's book verbal behavior. *The Analysis of Verbal Behavior, 9*, 81–96.

Sundberg, M. L. (1993). The application of establishing operations. *The Behavior Analyst, 16*, 211–214.

Sundberg, M. L. (2007). Verbal behavior. In J. O. Cooper, T. E. Heron, & W. L. Heward (Eds.), *Applied behavior analysis* (2nd ed., pp. 526–547). Upper Saddle River, NJ: Merrill/Prentice Hall.

Sundberg, M. L. (2008). *The verbal behavior milestones assessment and placement program: The VB-MAPP*. Concord, CA: AVB Press.

Sundberg, M. L. (2013). Thirty points about motivation from Skinner's book verbal behavior. *The Analysis of Verbal Behavior, 27*, 13–40.

Sundberg, M. L. (2014). *The verbal behavior milestones assessment and placement program: The VB-MAPP* (2nd ed.). Concord, CA: AVB Press.

Sundberg, M. L. (2015). The most important verbal operant. *VB News, 14*, 3–5.

Sundberg, M. L., Loeb, M., Hale, L., & Eigenheer, P. (2002). Contriving establishing operations to teach mands for information. *The Analysis of Verbal Behavior, 18*, 14–28.

Sundberg, M. L., & Michael, J. (2001). The benefits of Skinner's analysis of verbal behavior for children with autism. *Behavior Modification, 25*, 698–724.

Sundberg, M. L., Michael, J., Partington, J. W., & Sundberg, C. A. (1996). The role of automatic reinforcement in early language acquisition. *The Analysis of Verbal Behavior, 13*, 21–37.

Sundberg, M. L., Michael, J., & Peterson, N. (1977). Sign language: A behavioral analysis and applications. Kalamazoo MI: *Western Michigan University Behavioral Monograph #1*.

Sundberg, M. L., & Partington, J. W. (1998). *Teaching language to children with autism or other developmental disabilities*. Concord, CA: AVB Press.

Sundberg, M. L., & Partington, J. W. (1999). The need for both discrete trial and natural environment language training for children with autism. In P. M. Ghezzi, W. L. Williams, & J. E. Carr (Eds.), *Autism: Behavior analytic perspectives* (pp. 139–156). Reno, NV: Context Press.

Sundberg, M. L., & Sundberg, C. A. (2011). Intraverbal behavior and verbal conditional discriminations in typically developing children and children with autism. *The Analysis of Verbal Behavior, 27*, 23–43.

Touchette, P. E., & Howard, J. S. (1984). Errorless learning: Reinforcement contingencies and stimulus control transfer in delayed prompting. *Journal of Applied Behavior Analysis, 17*, 175–188.

Twyman, J. S. (1996). The functional independence of impure mands and tacts of abstract stimulus properties. *The Analysis of Verbal Behavior, 13*, 1–19.

Vaughan, M. E., & Michael, J. (1982). Automatic reinforcement: An important but ignored concept. *Behaviorism, 10*, 217–227.

Wallace, M. D., Iwata, B. A., & Hanley, G. P. (2006). Establishment of mands after tact training as a function of reinforcement strength. *Journal of Applied Behavior Analysis, 39*, 17–24.

Weiss, M. J., & Demiri, V. (2011). *Jumpstarting communication skills in children with autism*. Bethesda, MD: Woodbine House.

Wolf, M. M., Risley, T. R., & Mees, H. L. (1964). Application of operant controlling procedures to the behavior problems of an autistic child. *Behavior Research and Therapy, 1*, 305–312.

Wood, W. S., & Michael, J. (1977, May). *Special interest group: Teachers teaching courses using B. F. Skinner's book, Verbal Behavior (or, those who would like to).* Meeting held at the 3rd Annual Convention of the Midwestern Association for Behavior Analysis, Chicago, IL.

Wraikat, R., Sundberg, C. T., & Michael, J. (1991). Topography-based and selection-based verbal behavior: A further comparison. *The Analysis of Verbal Behavior, 9*, 1–17.

Yoon, S., & Bennett, G. M. (2000). Effects of a stimulus-stimulus pairing procedure on conditioning vocal sounds as reinforcers. *The Analysis of Verbal Behavior, 17*, 75–88.

Chapter 6
Panel Discussion

Raymond G. Romanczyk

Raymond G. Romanczyk: Now we are going to move into the next phase. All right, so just as a brief start to this, before we put all this together we had talked about as a group some common questions we are going to propose and the reference in your little brochure there, "A rose by any other name." The context is, as you can see, challenges to implementation. You all know that very well. It is one thing to know what to do; it is another to be able to have the resources to do it. If you build it, do you remember that phrase? Unfortunately, if you have evidence, they do not necessarily come. Right? Are evidence-based programs of the type you saw here, the norm or the exception in services? So it takes more than the evidence. Unfortunately, it is not sufficient. We do not live in a fully rational society. And it got me to thinking, all this nostalgia stuff looking at the old photos, when I was a graduate student at Rutgers University, a research project was done there that has influenced me my entire career and it was very simple. What they did is went to a little preschool, a campus preschool, and made some video tapes not unlike what you saw today and the study was very simple: take this one video tape of cute little kids in a teaching situation in a preschool. Two groups—the one group was told this is an example of a developmentally appropriate Montessori type of an event where children are encouraged to grow and they are nurtured by their therapist, etc.; the other group was told this is an example of behavior modification where individual skills are broken down into discrete units and taught in a sequence structure, blah, blah, blah… Then people were just asked where do you want to send you kid? I do not have to tell the results. They are very straightforward and they are very robust. How we describe things has great influence on consumers. Our purpose here today is very much instructional, but also to begin discussions. I do not want to use the word synthesis, that sounds too much like homogenization. It is more saying, "What are

R.G. Romanczyk (✉)
Institute for Child Development, Binghamton University,
Vestal Parkway East, Binghamton, NY 13902, USA
e-mail: rromanc@binghamton.edu

R.G. Romanczyk, J. McEachin (eds.), *Comprehensive Models of Autism Spectrum Disorder Treatment*, DOI 10.1007/978-3-319-40904-7_6

the commonalities? What are the things left to do?" And all the speakers talked about additional research we have to do. But as that takes place we have got to get implementation out there to so many kids and families in need. So we will start with some core questions to the panel and John, you are going to limit them, right? You are going to be my enforcer? What we are looking for is literally a 1–2 min response so we can get through a bunch and then we will get to audience questions. So if we start right to left. One of the questions was simply for all of you, what are the pragmatic challenges you face in implementation on getting services out to folks?

Ronald Leaf: I think staffing is a huge concern–having enough trained staff–and it is certainly a huge barrier. Funding is a barrier, as well. I think perhaps one of the biggest barriers is people not liking applied behavior analysis and having to change their conception of what that is and trying to separate out what it really is. I cannot tell you how many times I go to a conference where I hear, "I don't like ABA. I don't like what you do" and I ask back, "Well, what is that? What is ABA in your mind?" and I have to reframe it. We work with a lot of school districts. Clark County is actually the largest school district we work with in the country, and it started in a discussion with Charlene Green who was the superintendent and she said, "I am not going to use ABA in my schools." So I thought, "Why do you bring me here if you are going to use ABA?" but I said, "Well, what is ABA?" And she told me this horrendous story of ABA and had to acknowledge, "I don't like that either." So I think it is staffing, I think it is funding, I think it is a conception of what ABA is.

Sally Rogers: So I am not sure what getting it out means? If you mean how my group gets it out ourselves to the community, that is one issue. I guess for me, getting it out means giving it to other people to use. How do I disseminate it? How do we make it scalable to folks in the 0–3 systems, even within the most limited 0–3 service deliveries that there are? And how do we put something that is more effective than what is going on in the hands of people who have very little time and very little training and very little autism expertise? And I am trying to do that. I am trying to figure out how to do that right now, but I think there are several things. I do not know what the core elements are. I know that there are a lot of collateral effects with each of the interventions that we do. I have not had a chance to study those, break it down, and figure out what are the essential pieces. That is one problem, when we do teach it in community settings—how to get people to have time to practice, time to actually try it, time to score themselves, time to think, time to have peer supervision. This is highly technical intervention and particularly in the beginning before it becomes automatic, it requires a lot of thought and a lot of time, and that is very precious in the understaffed public settings. I am always thinking about public settings. How to create enough trainers—we have a huge demand and it takes a couple of years for us to start with somebody and have them at a point where they really can train other people and so the supply, all of those are huge barriers for me.

Mark L. Sundberg: Well, I agree with everything that has been said so far. It is hard stuff, but here is an addition to what they said. We are not getting much help at the college level. I mean, we really need to have behavior analysis in special education programs, speech pathology programs, at the high school level. My kids took a psychology class in high school and a standard textbook, which is a survey course on behavior analysis, and they basically slander behavior analysis. I mean here are 14, 15, 16-year-old kids and look at the content that is in those textbooks. It is very inaccurate, often. But, again, I do not think we have gotten buy-in from special education departments—we have got a few places like Gonzaga and Ohio State—but yet for the most part, this, as the previous two speakers said, this is hard stuff and it is not something that you want to do after somebody already has a degree; it needs to get into the college curriculum.

William Ahearn: Well I was talking about how NECC has established systems for distributing our expertise and, if I was going to pick one thing, which I will not, I would say it's time. It has taken an enormous amount of time to put together the systems to be able to bring our systems to scale, but we have done it. If I was going to pick number two it is to have people that can effectively communicate about what it is that they are doing and if I am going to give a third one, I would take some time to very clearly state that the majority of people who do behavior analysis are not psychologists. The majority of them out there are education-based people and people that have specialties in behavior analysis. I wish that Skinner's radical behaviorism had been adopted in psychology as a problem and an approach, but it was not and as Mark said, the problem is that the way you are going to encounter behavior analysis in psychology, in general, is in a way that looks at it with a negative light.

Raymond G. Romanczyk: It is sort of a common theme there in terms of perception. Next one for everyone, what is the approximate cost per child per year and the typical source of funding for the child?

Ronald Leaf: There is obviously a range in our cost and it depends upon the intensity of the intervention, but I would say our standard intervention is 30 h weekly that children are receiving, 12 h of supervision monthly, and 2 h of psychologist time per month, so that is our standard and that is around $120,000 for the year. We have less and more, but that would be standard case. In terms of funding, our funding is primarily insurance and school districts. That would be the funding source for us. I think we have one private pay, maybe two private pay clients, and that is in our office in Los Angeles. In our other offices internationally, it is much less and the funding is primarily private pay.

Sally Rogers: I showed that to you in a slide, but I did not actually read what the slide said, when I showed the cost benefit analysis. I think David Mandel figured that he was somewhere around $50,000 a year for the UW site and most of the work I do is inside research protocols, so in our particular site, we are not serving kids publicly very much. Other people who are using ESDM are doing a lot of public services, but my group does not, so I do not really price it for my area.

Mark L. Sundberg: I unfortunately do not really have an answer to the question. I do not work within a program or an agency per se like the other three. Primarily, I have been in the public schools for the last 10 years and, basically, it costs way more than they want to pay. We just had an administrator say, "Back in my day, we had 20 kids and only a teacher and an aide. Why can't you do that?" You know, and that is the mentality that we struggle within the public school system.

William Ahearn: Okay, so in terms of costs relative to early intensive behavioral intervention for a home-based service in Massachusetts, which is paid through the state education system, it is a very interesting cost share. The best thing that ever happened in Massachusetts—thank you very much, Autism Speaks—was passing autism insurance reform, which eventually led to the ditching of the early intervention services that were in place and the reestablishing of the services that the state took over and that allowed us to provide services that were not money losers. So currently, our home-based services are about $1500 a week, so when we translate that into a year, we are talking $75,000–80,000 a year. That is for our services. Our services are much more expensive than a number of others. If it was private paying, it would be more. Our intensive instruction program, remember that is the day services, a 226-day a year program. It is about $100,000 for those that are being paid for in-state. There are a number of sort permutations with that but the most that it could cost would be $120,000 a year, for private payers. For residential services, remember this is the severe problem behavior, 24 h care, and primarily one to one and sometimes greater staffing ratios, we are talking about $208,000 a year up to $257,000 a year. Our staff intensive, those are intractable problem behavior kids that come in, are about $316,000 a year starting and ranging up to private paying $391,000. And we have a very small adult services program which is an incredible money loser much less than that, but we keep that in place mainly to be in that system and serving some of our kids that have become young adults.

Raymond G. Romanczyk: The next questions folks really did touch on, I think, and we are going to focus on the latter half of this question: the role of parents and caregivers in intervention, and moreover, what support and services do they receive in the programs?

Ronald Leaf: As I said in my presentation, parent buy-in and expertise is essential in our program and that there are many kinds of services our parents receive: they receive parent training to deal with not only the everyday issues, sleep issues, eating issues, whatever is occurring, also to help generalize what we are doing in the services we do and that is one level of service for our parents. We also offer, for our parents, therapy. Often, our parents are receiving therapeutic supports, dealing with grieving, kinds of issues, marital issues that come out of it, whatever really is affecting the family. We are dealing with that as well. We also do sibling groups too, so that is what our resources are.

Sally Rogers: As I said, parents who are getting intensive services for their child get a parent coaching session every other week; one is in the center and one is at home. We have a specific protocol that we use. We are influenced by Hanf, Rush, and Sheldon model of coaching. Parents really like that approach a lot. We also use motivational interviewing and stages of change, in terms of our thoughts with them. We teach them to use the interactive principles of ESDM and we work with them to build them into their daily routines at home and in the community with other children. We do not ask them to keep data, we do not expect them to keep data—although some do and some want to—and we have a parent manual, which we have both written and multimedia ways for them to access it, and it has a curriculum that we use with them. We also provide referrals as they need them for other services—

any kind of services they need, particularly in the field of mental health. We make sure that they are tied into family advocacy groups that are in the area. We refer them to our regional center for support groups.

Mark L. Sundberg: I think it is pretty clear that the more that the parents are involved and know, the better progress the child is going to make, but it is not necessarily just involvement. That is, that we have parents that are very involved and cause more problems, so it is proactively involved. You know, just as a humor note Dick Malott has a concept that he calls *pissed-off autism mammas*. If you have ever seen Dick Malott give that talk, it is pretty hilarious, and he makes the point that so much of what is happened in our field is because of parents and that we look at and he gives examples people like Mary Barbera, who is a parent of child with autism and has written books and a variety of other people that have certainly helped us a lot. Parents make a huge difference and we should get them on board early. I try to make the case that we do not want to sit down with parents at the IEP for the first time. They need to be coming to the classroom. We need to teach them as much as we can. They have got to be involved, for a variety of reasons—I will just give you two real quick ones: in terms of language training and motivating operations that are available in the evenings and weekends and all kinds of other settings, especially aversive motivators, the "I don't want to take a bath, I don't want to put my shoes on, I don't want to get in the car seat, I don't want to leave the video game." How do you deal with those? We do not have those problems necessarily in an academic or a classroom setting because of control of the video in various ways, so a lot of the problems that a parent faces, we do not have in a controlled educational setting. The discriminative stimuli that occur in a typical environment, in the parents' environment, are not the same that we have in a classroom. We have got a very, kind of sterile environment. There are only so many boxes of materials, yet the natural environment is loaded with all kinds of different antecedents that, if we can teach the parent how to do mand, tact and intraverbal training, how to get rid of behavior problems, and so on, it is only going to help us as a team.

William Ahearn: Just to reflect what the other three have said, certainly parent involvement is critical to optimal outcome and home-based services is obviously somewhat different, since you are there all the time with the parent. We set out what our goals are in monthly clinics that are with the parents, where there is no service being provided. The expert level supervision of the case is meeting with the parent for 1 h every month and setting out the priorities, and then for the home-based kids, on a daily basis; for those in day services, so anyone still living at home, there is a weekly 1-h session in which the teachers go in and work with the parent to implement what the primary objectives are usually from the parent's perspective, whatever the biggest problem is.

Ronald Leaf: If I can just add, I think I took like 20 s, so can I take two more minutes? I think it starts with understanding what parents go through as best we can: the dilemma, the nightmare they live every day, from the very beginning when mom knows there is something wrong and everyone is saying no it is not, there is nothing wrong. Pediatricians say no you are an overanxious mom, you are not doing it or you are doing too much and they have to face that so early on and then they enter into the school system and usually it is an adversarial relationship from the very get-go, when you think of the IEPs across this country. This side is parents; this side is school. And often times it is in a condescending way to parents and we need to understand what they are going through the best we can. I do not have a child with autism. I have been doing this a long time, but I try to connect the best I can and understand their dilemma and challenge and set up that connection so that then we can go on and do the work that needs to be done. It is just recognizing the massive challenge they go through.

Raymond G. Romanczyk: To underscore that, there is clear literature out there that the families of children with autism are under much higher stress than families with children with other disorders, physical, emotional, etc. It is an under-researched area for those of you out there still working those theses. All right. Replication, what is the feasibility of your model being fully implemented by other service agents? It is not meant as a trick question, it is really where are you at this stage in dissemination?

Ronald Leaf: For us, replication… we have I think nine offices within our agency and it is replicated across all nine offices. Fidelity, doing the same work that we are doing in our home office. Replication, there are other agencies that are not our agencies that we are working with and helping train and seeing very similar results with the same methodology being used. Our largest replication—we work with schools across the country. I consider what we do sort of the Ferrari model perhaps, but we cannot do that in schools. In schools, it is sort of a Chevrolet. I mean that is what the law really states and that is what we have to make happen, so we are working with aides, teachers, everyone that touches a child's life, and trying to get them to do very similar things. They are not going to be identical things, but it is quite similar. As I look at these three folks [present today] from Clark county that we have worked with for years, they do amazing work here but unfortunately it's not throughout the system. There are problems within the system, it's the largest school district, but we are replicating what we do in our office in large part in schools. And as Sally's talked about, we have got to be able to provide that kind of service. It has to be economical. It has to be feasible and so we have learned how to take our model and how to work with, you know, aides that have no training whatsoever and get them on board.

Sally Rogers: I think there is a difference between replication and dissemination. In terms of replication, we have multiple sites that replicate our model fully. They are research sites. We go through all kinds of procedures to make sure everybody is doing things the same and data systems and things like that. And we have university settings, multiple ones in the world right now to have set up ESDM and are doing research, we have a University in Australia, there is one in Italy, there is a group in France, there is a group in Canada, Vanderbilt University, Cornell… so we have got replications. We also have sites that have taken on ESDM as a clinical model offering services privately. They learn it; they do it. I do not follow it. I hear about it, but it is not a databased system, so I have no idea how well fidelity is maintain. I know the state of Maine has taken on ESDM as their 0–3 model. I think Nevada wants to do that, as well. Easter Seals in California says they do ESDM and they have a contract with one of the big insurers. I have no idea how much ESDM training has actually gone on there. So I mean, when you train, you turn things loose and you are really dependent on people to be honest about what they are doing and it is also why we publish on our website the name of every person that is certified and every level that they been certified across the world and how to reach them, so that consumers have some access to training and services from people that we have trained. I think another challenge for this and for scalability is motivating the people who are out there to use it. It is more difficult to do ESDM than to do what is typically out there in the low-intensity 0–3 systems. It requires more from adults and I do not know that they work as well. And I do not know if the reinforcement systems that I experience when I work with children are in place for the people who are doing one visit every 2 weeks in the woods of Idaho with a difficult family and a hard child and trying to help the parent do ESDM there. I do not know how to build the motivation in for those folks to go through the effort that it takes. It is one of the things we have got to figure out.

Mark L. Sundberg: Following up on Sally's point, it is the word *fully* in there that makes it a little difficult in our field. Successive approximations are something that is very important to us and I think that looking at all the skills we have talked about, to be able to fully implement all the political variables, there are a lot of obstacles and barriers to doing this and that is where we are happy with successive approximations in various kinds of settings. We are glad to see them take data, reinforce, stop reinforcing problem behaviors, and so there is a lot of work. I would like to give you two examples of replication. The first is the Behavior Analysis Center for Autism which is operated by Carl and Devon Sundberg, (yes that is my brother and sister-in-law) and I am keeping it in the family, but yeah over the last 4 or 5 years, they have developed four programs around Indianapolis that replicate the Verbal Behavior model. It is a lot of work. I am involved in their program and it is a nonstop staff training type project and I think there are something like 244 employees. Same with Autism Partnership, you guys have a lot of people that have to be trained and it is hard to keep up with and requires a lot of skill. The second model, in the state of Pennsylvania, the Pennsylvania Technical Training and Assistance Network operated by the Department of Education in the state of Pennsylvania funds the PaTTAN Autism Initiative. They began 15 years ago, implementing a verbal behavior model in one classroom supervised by a guy named Mike Miklos. I got an email from Mike this morning. Mike is now director of the whole program. He said they are now up to 460 classrooms around the state of Pennsylvania that are using the verbal behavior model. They have a very sophisticated criterion in order to receive the funding, the support. They employ, not as many as Bill, but I think they have about 50 BCBAs, which is essential and, again, this is in the public school setting. They presented data of 800 VB-MAPPs on their kids from preschool to high school age. It has been a labor of love for these guys. They have fought political battles and so on, but yet the program is growing.

William Ahearn: It would probably be twice the number of classrooms in Pennsylvania, if they had not so screwed up the qualifications for identifying people and if they set the BACB criteria, they would be much further along then. It was harder to become behavior specialists with BACB criteria than it was if you were an occupational therapist who took one workshop from someone who says that they are a behavioral analyst and without credentials. I could go on and on state by state as to what the issues are, but in terms of, one of the things that has been kind of interesting and some of it is just happenstance, replications of our model have happened. Some of our scaling has actually been up. The resources that go to providing services to the kids in our school Abu Dhabi… you know we here in the United States are jealous with the amount of resources and the amount of space available for working with individuals over there and being able to bring to scale our model involved very careful planning and some of it was fairly straightforward. You want to be able to translate what you are doing from English alone to make sure that it is Arabic, to eventually build up a large percentage of your staff, so that the majority of the staff are Arabic speakers, so all of what it took to go to scale there was relatively easy to plan for. Going the other direction is much more difficult, so scaling out into the public and private schools that are using our models of service delivery, really the biggest challenges are having expertise and skill acquisition. We can provide help or at least bring other people in for working with problem behavior, but to be able to implement the systems for establishing skills, there really needs to be some level of expertise on the floor with respect to skill acquisition and staff training. They are the two biggest obstacles. In terms of being able to go from the intensity of service, there certainly is a trade-off. The fewer resources you have to bring, the less of the gains are. One of the ways we have been attempting to bring our model to scale, more and more economically, is by constant end-user survey, to try to make it easier, meet the challenges that are occurring in the different environments in which our model is being used.

Raymond G. Romanczyk: This next one come from the speakers themselves in a sense with their very frequent references to food and eating related activities and that is the analogy of *recipes*. We have talked about the distinction within training programs of cooking versus baking. Cooking, flair, innovation, changes, substitutions—baking, you do that and what happens? Baking is precise measurement, specific ratios, specific ingredients, specific times, all that good stuff. So the question is, in the context of your program, in a very loose kind of way what ratio would you think is cooking versus baking? You start out with the recipes.

Ronald Leaf: Yes, I am lost with that one; I just switched my spaghetti sauce that Tony [Cuvo] taught me to make and I am thinking about that. So if I understand, cooking is flair and innovation, while baking is standardized precision. Does that mean we are protocol driven when we are baking? So baking a cake you have to follow the recipe? Well, I do not know I agree with that level of thinking, but nonetheless my wife is an incredible baker and she changes things and the taste of things; so I think it is a combination. We have a map that we use and that is the precision part of it and we train to precision and so we do some baking, I guess. We alter that all the time too. I cannot give you an exact percent, I am going to say maybe 65–75 % cooking… I cannot tell you. It is a blend, an absolute blend and we do get our research published, so we have protocols that we have to follow, otherwise we would not have the publications we have got but we have to define very clearly what baking is and what cooking is. I am going to end up saying 90–10; 90 % we cook, 10 % we bake. John is saying now 80–20. Because if there are five of us, the five psychologists that all came from UCLA, we do it five different ways. But I am sticking with 90–10.

Sally Rogers: I am not going to talk about cooking and baking. I am talking about degrees of freedom and I think, I actually feel like ESDM is an extremely creative approach to treatment, in that the therapist—and this is one of the burdens of it—the therapist has a responsibility of deciding what is going to be taught from the curriculum, so you have got a structure for looking at things. The curriculum kind of lays out the skill set, but it is up to the therapist to make the decisions, to form those objectives, to break them down in the way they are going to teach them, and then you walk into every session and there is absolutely no script. There are just activities, which you create with the child together, and other than having materials around the room that you know are going to get you to certain objectives, what you do in that hour is really yours and it is the chemistry of you and child and the parent and the moment with materials and whatever arousal state everybody's in, so I feel like, kind of the rules, like teach multiple objectives in each activity and build these four-part routines, they give kind of a structure to the time and a structure what you are doing, but nothing tells you what to do in the moment or with the child and so I think for clinicians, for people like all of us who spent lots of time with the kids, it is really nice to be able to do this because it does let you use clinical judgment and all of your clinical skills in what is happening, but the framework also makes it easier for new people to step into this. It gives them a lot of rules about how to build something, so that they know where to start. So I feel like the structure allows for a great range of individuality and degrees of freedom within it. But without the structure, it would be a disorganized mess and you would not be able to get where you want to go.

Mark L. Sundberg: Skinner wrote a paper called *A Case History in Scientific Method* about 50 years ago and, in that paper, he made several points, one of which was, if you run into something interesting drop everything else and study it. And there was a psychologist named Willard Day–does anybody in the audience know who Willard Day was? Willard Day had a methodology he called *radical methodology* and part of the point of radical methodology and its connections to Skinner's paper was that independent variables occur in our day-to-day interaction that were not planned, not programmed, motivating operations that occur that are not in our script. And if we sit down with kids, the kids are responding to our questions. They are giving us behavior, they are presenting independent variables that we could not have not predicted might have occurred prior to beginning of the session. We might go in with a script. We say to a kid what do you like to eat and he says chow mein, ok, so now all of a sudden chow mein becomes a verbal discriminative stimulus for me that is going to have something to do with my next question. Now if I look down and say very good tell me an animal, it is like whoa wait a minute I thought we were talking about chow mein and I think a lot of times people go in with a scripted kind of program. Our staff used to always want me to script the correction procedure and I refused to do it and Stacy's laughing because you remember our argument about this 15 or 20 years ago. What exactly do I do when there is an error? And I always say that it depends. The staff needed to know exactly what to do. Well there are advantages to some degree. You have got to have some of that in there, some very clear cut kind of general pattern, but there has to be room for subject- or client- or child-generated independent variables that affect your behavior as a scientist, a clinician, and such. And I do not think they can be ignored, so it is a combination, and Bill is going to have a comment, I can just tell.

William Ahearn: Yeah I love project A, just like Skinner did, and if you know anything about a *Case History in Scientific Method*, I am lying through my teeth. The task he was given by project A was to describe his operationism and essentially Skinner's response was like giving everybody the finger. So he said essentially control your conditions was the first point and he says that it was Pavlov that taught him how important that was and then he goes into all of these other points like, serendipity—drop everything. When we find something interesting, drop everything else and study that. He also says some people are lucky. No they are not lucky. You get lucky perhaps every once in a while, when you are working hard and you prepared, then you can take advantage of those situation in which something spurious happens. He also says that part of what is very important to operationism is to be lazy, so that is how we discovered intermittent reinforcement because he wanted to go out on the weekend and did not want to spend all weekend putting together food pellets for the pigeon and the rats. So when I take a look at this question, this is the stupidest question ever asked, who asked this question? It was us. Well, it was the most brilliant question I have ever heard. In some ways it is difficult to come up with—I liked how you struggled and started with one level of percentage then another because it is really—those two things do not work up against one another. They are together. With your precision, with your protocols, there needs to be flexibility. Where is your flexibility? Your flexibility is within the implementation of the teaching procedures. What do I want my teachers to do? Do I want them to take what they have learned in their course work and then go work with kids? Hell no, that does not work. I want them to act like me or the other people that are providing treatment. That is the model and that is Skinner's point in the case history. How one becomes a scientist is not by taking classes, it is by being a scientist and engaging in scientific behavior. One needs to be of the same mindset when it comes to clinical application. It is very important to very precisely control your conditions and to be flexible with respect to teaching procedures—to evaluate what is going on in front of you and being able to change on the fly is very important at times and at other times, it is very important to not change on the fly because you need to be patient and wait for that opportune moment to happen. It is not always on the first trial and if you start something else, you might find that you never get what you wanted to get in the first place but you would have if you would have stuck with where you started, so you know I am going to not answer the question.

Raymond G. Romanczyk: I think they all answered our core questions very well. Now, we are going to switch just a little. John, do you want to come on up?

Chapter 7
Commentary on Commonalities and Divergence

John McEachin

John McEachin: I have attempted to categorize some commonalities and possible points of divergence across the models. Let's start with what these four models share in common. These are my thoughts:

Commonalities

1. They have a strong ethic on being data-driven and making decisions that are based on objective data.
2. All four are informed by a learning/behavioral theory of one type or another.
3. All four incorporate a developmental model to some extent.
4. Each is aimed at remediating important skill deficits and replacing detrimental behavior with more adaptive behavior.
5. I think we can say they are all ambitious in what they aim to accomplish.
6. Similarly, they all seem to be comprehensive in scope.

We can see different flavors of behaviorism and different branches of the behavioral family tree represented here, e.g. Watson and Thorndike vs. Skinner and radical behaviorism vs. a more pragmatic type of behaviorism, but the models are all informed by learning theory, including the ESDM model.

Developmental theory is present most clearly in the ESDM model, but in the other three models we can also see evidence of the practitioners respecting the fact that the children are able to do certain skills at one age and other skills not until an older age. In the evolution of intensive behavioral programs for young children with autism, we didn't start out explicitly investigating developmental sequence, but the mere fact that practitioners were responsive to the success and failures of their work meant that they were moving up and down the developmental hierarchy, ultimately

J. McEachin (✉)
Autism Partnership, 200 Marina Drive, Seal Beach, CA 90740, USA
e-mail: JMAutPar@aol.com

R.G. Romanczyk, J. McEachin (eds.), *Comprehensive Models of Autism Spectrum Disorder Treatment*, DOI 10.1007/978-3-319-40904-7_7

being shaped into adhering to a developmental model. The quicker we figured out the importance of the developmental model, the more successful we were.

I do think it's fair to say that we can identify certain behaviors that kids on the spectrum engage in as being detrimental and these are four examples of models that are aiming very explicitly to try to steer kids away from behaviors that would be detrimental and to promote an expansion of a repertoire of behaviors that we would regard as adaptive. We can talk in a minute about where the models diverge in terms of directiveness, but even Sally's child-centered model seems to care about discouraging detrimental behavior.

I'm pretty sure that we can see aspirations toward being comprehensive, although Mark talked a little bit more about the verbal behavior repertoire of individuals. However, I do know that, within the work that Mark does, they are aiming to cover more than just language skills.

Differences

1. Subtype of behavioral model and inclusion of theories beyond a strictly behavioral approach.
2. Parental involvement?
3. The entry point for starting programming and choosing curricular targets.
4. Aiming for replicability and manualization of the model
5. Willingness and readiness to be directive
6. Centrality of Skinner's analysis of verbal behavior
7. Research informing versus driving clinical practice
8. Adults as mediators of social contingencies
9. A relative emphasis on group versus one-to-one

Particularly with respect to the ESDM model, we can see a difference in some specific theoretical approaches that inform the work. Sally's model is not as exclusively reliant on behavioral theory.

It would appear that settings is not an important factor in driving outcomes, but rather more a reflection of real-world practicality. For example, the NEC model happens to be in a school, but very likely, the fact that it's in the school isn't an essential part of the model.

Parental involvement? I'm not sure about this and perhaps the presenters could address the extent to which they consider parents to be integrally involved. In Sally's model, it's very explicit. In Bill's model, it seems to not be explicitly incorporated.

In service delivery models for children with ASD, there is a continuum of degree of structuredness and willingness to contrive opportunities to practice the skill versus, at the other end of the continuum, a more naturalistic, incidental teaching approach. I think within the four models described here, everyone aspires to move toward as naturalistic as possible, but I suspect that there are differences within the models about where they are more likely to start as the entry point on that continuum.

The aim for replicability and manualization of the model is prominent in Sally's description of the ESDM model. She seems to be explicitly aiming to come up with a model that can be manualized and widely implemented without decades of apprenticeship before being willing to let people have a go at it. And I'd probably put Ron at the other end of that continuum.

On willingness and readiness to be directive, I think there are differences; I'm going to leave that to each of you to make a comment on.

And, of course, specifically with Mark's presentation, the centrality of Skinner's analysis of verbal behavior is central to the model.

On the dimension of research informing versus driving clinical practice, I think this is little bit like the idea of protocol-driven versus flexible. The NEC model seemed to be at the protocol-driven end of the spectrum, while the Autism Partnership/Lovaas model is on the other end of the spectrum.

What about adults as mediators of social contingencies within the learning opportunities that students get? Perhaps the speakers can touch on where their model falls on the continuum.

So let me turn it over to the presenters to comment on differences and commonalities as they see them.

Ahearn: Sure, I'll start with learning theory because I'm a trained learning theorist. I think I'm the only one up here who is a trained learning theorist in experimental psychology and I sort of start with Skinner's approach as informing what we should think of learning theory and I think it would be a farce to all together do away with theory. If I'm directly quoting, it's not the intent, it's just the number of times that I've read, "Are theories of learning necessary?" And the essential point of it is that, if we are talking about something occurring in some other dimension, that learning theory is not very useful. If we are talking about learning as we see it, observe it, and measure over time what's happening, a very careful inductive process may lead us to generalizations, deductions, that come from that origin of a very careful induction prior to developing some grand theory. It's very important because what we lose with respect to that is what is learned and that is behavior. So when I think of learning theory and, as I just said, I was trained in learning theory, from Watson to Hull to Miller and Dollard and the majority of the reason why I have this notion that learning theory is not particularly useful, it's because I don't feel it's scientific. When we talk about theory, per se, should we be looking for that? Yes, but that's different and that's Skinner's points in "are theories of learning necessary?" When we posit that there is something in some other dimension, but we can't touch it, then that's not science. If we are talking about what we see and we stick with the things unto themselves, we will be able to move to more and more complex subject matter without making the errors that hypothesis-driven experimentation has led to the cyclical breaking down of systems within psychology and rebuilding new ones. That has been the history, at least in the United States, in psychology. So I would say I differ greatly in that I think that theories of learning are not necessary, but what we need are theories, like if we want to talk about theories of autism, I've posited one, embedded within what I was talking about, a social learning disorder is what autism is, starting from the very initial differences and that informs our practice very differently than if we were just assuming that, well, this is something that is organic within the individual and we are kind of just going to have cobble on a way of producing some new executive function where there was executive dysfunction and that's not useful. What is useful is starting with where the individual is. When I see how practice is very well informed by what the contributions of autism research broadly have brought, in that we have a very keen understanding from careful research that has identified what's different in individuals with autism, as opposed to what's different in typically developing and other developmental disabilities, which has led to a flurry of research relative to what does this mean, how does it translate across the lifespan, and what is effective for meeting these particular objectives? Because clinical application is two steps removed from scientific investigation. So, I stop now.

McEachin: I think it was poor choice of words on my part. I take from what you are saying that you would be happier with "informed by behavioral theory" or the scientific method.

Sundberg: Well, of the many topics I'll pick one or two. Structured teaching versus natural environment teaching and that whole issue. In the late '70s and early '80s, Bob Koegel and colleagues kind of started this whole line of research that natural environment or the pivotal response model is far better than Lovaas' structured teaching kind of model and there is a number of studies that came out that attempted to demonstrate that and the issue is that two different things were being compared in that line of research. That is, mand training, for example, is nicely done in a natural environment where natural motivators occur and there is much to be gained in the natural environment. Other skills, though, are much better taught in a structured teaching session. For example, if you are doing matching to sample or tacting, it's nice to be able to have available to you, at a table, multiple exemplars, big and little items, all kinds of materials you simply cannot find in the natural environment. So the whole notion that you can just do natural environment training really doesn't work in my mind. You need that blend of both careful, structured, systematic teaching, which is really where the kids are going to go anyway if they are going to make it into less restrictive settings. When they get into a classroom, they will be doing tabletop activities. They will have worksheets. There will be discrete trial activities, such as "do these ten math problems". You cannot follow a kid's EO all the time. If you have ten kids, you cannot get down on the floor with them whenever they want and play with whatever item that they want. While it's a useful procedure, I don't think it's a methodology that we want to say we are going to endorse full force. We will take the parts of it that are valuable, but we also need structured teaching.

McEachin: Thanks Mark. Can I just quickly ask, the video clip that you showed there, would you regard that as NET?

Sundberg: No that was very, very contrived. In fact, it was very mass trial. I only did manding. It was single trial in a controlled setting, very structured kind of interaction. Now if I were to get into NET, staying away from the table and being in other kinds of settings, I would want to see if I can get this child to mand for candy—having first established the skill in a controlled setting. Only then would I begin to move in others ways. I would not probably have been able to establish this skill solely in the natural environment. I need instructional control. See that was a kid who liked to bolt and nobody could get him to sit down and you saw, in one trial, I'm bringing him back and as soon as he failed he was turning to bolt and a so controlled teaching arrangement is very valuable and I think that's an element of structured teaching. I'm not going to follow his EOs all the time. That's just not the way it works. Try that as a parent with your typical kids. You will quickly find yourself saying "I'm sorry we are not doing that now."

McEachin: I feel a theme emerging here. Sally?

Rogers: Okay, well it's clear I'm kind of the outsider in some ways, not just gender. So I'm just going to say what I think. First of all, the idea that instructional control requires structured teaching… I don't think that is necessary. I think you can have instructional control. You can have it at a dinner table. You can have it when you have the ball. It doesn't require the child sitting in a chair being at a table to have instructional control. I think that's what PRT and incidental teaching approaches have shown us. You have instructional control as soon as you control the goal that the child has. That's how you get control. So I don't think those two things necessarily go together. It's easier to get the attention of children when there's nothing there and you've got their bodies contained. I guess, when I think about the importance of structure and structured teaching, I've always had a problem with TEACCH because of this, I think about the arguments that people have about the introduction of too much structure in academic teaching in typical preschools and how much we think about how sitting down and attending to an adult and learning through verbal mechanisms isn't necessarily the best way to teach young children anything. It's a model that people, particularly Europeans, don't approve at all. The hands on learning model fits young children's learning and that's accepted anywhere and I think the idea that children with autism need something different because they are different kinds of learners, I don't know that we have the evidence that we think we do for that. You know, it used to be that people thought, "Why would I use a developmental model, there's no data that children with autism follow normal developmental trajectories", but lo and behold, there is plenty of evidence that children with autism follow developmental trajectories. We think that they're all visual learners. Well, you know they are not all visual learners. There is a whole range of learning styles, so I think the assumption that children with autism need a different learning approach is one that is not necessarily supported by science. So I think that there are preferences, but I don't know that you need a certain amount of physical control over a child's body in order to get their attention or to teach them a new skill and I think the younger they are, the more likely it is that you are going to have fewer learning opportunities. The more you require inhibition, sitting, and doing nothing, you are going to lose a lot of time in delivering learning opportunities. So I think there is not one best way to do any of these things. I guess there are a couple of other differences I saw that I wanted to throw on the table. I think there are big differences in the way teaching targets are chosen and, for me, it's really important that the teaching targets are meaningful to the child and the child's own life and their own goals, that they fit the contexts within which the children are learning, and when you just gave the example of needing cards at the table because maybe the objects you want to build in the child's vocabulary wasn't in the child's environment, I would say, "well, if those objects aren't in the child's environment, why do they need the words for those?" They need the words for the things that are their environment. That's what we all talk about. It isn't until we are in school that we learn the names of things that we don't act on a daily basis. So I think this issue of ecological fittedness, meaningfulness, how much of this goal is the child going to understand, is it useful, is it relevant to their moment-to-moment lives and interactions… I think that's a big difference across approaches. I think another big difference is the way that we characterize the nature of the adult's behavior towards the child. You know, I talked about affect and warmth and sensitivity and responsivity to children's cues and I think that is an area actually where there is a lot of agreement in terms of your idea—playfulness, warmth, enjoyment of the child, expressing the pleasure that we feel, making an environment in which the kids are not afraid of us, they want to be interacting. But it's not explicit in other therapies that I know about from a behavioral tradition. People talk about and you see these qualities and you know that makes good teachers, but I don't see it in the fidelity systems that are coming from these and you might find it useful to put them in because I think it's a commonality in practice, but I don't see a language for it in some of the other approaches.

Ahearn: I want to say something that is in complete agreement. The education system in the United States is completely broken.

Leaf: Back to Ray's question earlier about cooking vs. baking. Yes, yes, yes, and yes. I think it was 85–15 now that I think about it, and I make great cinnamon rolls, by the way, like they're amazing. But you have to see when they are golden. Sometimes it's 25 min; sometimes it's 35 min. You never quite know. There's an art to knowing when they are ready to go. Yes, yes, yes, and yes, back to that one. By the way, Bill, my PhD was in learning, so I'm a learning theorist, too. I was influenced by all the people you said and Guthrie and Estes and Hull and all those folks. I think it's the backbone of what we do. I took what they did and learned from that and adapted. I don't really think about what we do in theoretical terms. Whenever I start to think I have it figured out, at the end of the day, I realize I don't. I'm not as smart as these three at all. I don't understand what they are saying some of the time. I just take kids, we look at what they need, and we just figure it out. For me it's a continuum of structure. It's from naturalistic to restrictive and everything in between, artificial and natural and we take a kid and say, "Let's try this one. Let's try to be more natural and see what happens." We probe and take data. If we aren't happy with the results then okay, let's be a little more structured. The term we would use, John doesn't like this term, but structured flexibility is a term we have used for I think 20 years, meaning there is a structure but we're flexible within that structure and I don't know if it's a learning theory or behavioral theory or whose theory we're following, we just work with kids. And, again, at the end of the day, we train staff. We train staff in schools, and in our agency, and they can do it too. What they mostly need is to be a critical thinker, probing, and quickly recognize when things are changing. That's what we do.

McEachin: Something I think is important to say here is that, in listening to Sally and the others, you can hear that there are hypotheses about what makes a difference and what doesn't make a difference. We have four models where we have clear empirical evidence that, following this model, positive results can be obtained with children. The thing is, we haven't done the component analyses and, although it would be very difficult to do, we really need to do more of that. All of us who do this work, all of us in this room here, we have hypotheses that we adhere to, that we consider very dear, about what are the components that we think are essential. We see the change and we attribute the change to things that we do, but we don't actually know that the thing we are attributing it to is actually responsible for the change. So all of the things Sally said are testable hypotheses and, if in fact, by conceptualizing what you do in a more developmental humanistic way, gets you better results, let's find that out or let's find out for which kids would this approach be better or not better. There are many things that each of these practitioners does every day that are not necessarily described as an integral part of their model, not necessarily conceptualized, but may still make a significant contribution to the overall package. Attempting to replicate without including these essential pieces would not work as well.

And I think, with that, we need to let the audience ask some questions.

Chapter 8
Audience Questions and Closing Comments

Raymond G. Romanczyk

Audience question read by Raymond G. Romanczyk: This is to all the presenters, "What sort of success rates have you had for your models in achieving insurance reimbursement for your services?". That's a pragmatic question.

Ronald Leaf: I'm looking at Andy who's not looking at me, who does our insurance. I think we are really successful. I think most of our kids are funded through insurance. Julie McEachin has done amazing job in insurance. We get funded for insurance, so it's been, I wouldn't say easy, but it's happened. It depends what kind of insurance the parents have. And what state. Like California.

Sally Rogers: There are people using ESDM who do get insurance reimbursement. We don't get insurance reimbursement right now through the hospital because the staffing patterns that we use aren't medically billable, so we are in the middle of that right now and I'm trying to figure out the solutions to that, but other people are getting reimbursed for ESDM.

Mark L. Sundberg: I want to see if I can get my brother to answer. You're on the spot, or your wife. We are in Midwest and I'd really encourage people to get in touch with Autism Speaks because they really connect to people all over the US and there is just a variety of different reasons why you may or may not get these claims covered.

William Ahearn: We don't do insurance reimbursed work except for in our home-based services. In the state of Massachusetts, we have a very strong division of insurance, which has implemented insurance reform mandate in a way that is working for the practitioners on the ground, which is why the number of behavioral analysts is increasing exponentially in Massachusetts—the greatest number of per capita behavioral analyst in the world. But really, insurance reimbursement is something that is about to become a real challenge if the CPT codes that were developed

R.G. Romanczyk (✉)
Institute for Child Development, Binghamton University, Vestal Parkway East, Binghamton, NY 13902, USA
e-mail: rromanc@binghamton.edu

R.G. Romanczyk, J. McEachin (eds.), *Comprehensive Models of Autism Spectrum Disorder Treatment*, DOI 10.1007/978-3-319-40904-7_8

ABAI which are just an abysmal nightmare because they don't include supervision and if, by the way, if you are member ABAI, please fill out the practitioner survey that probably hit your email inbox today to let them know that there needs to be supervision codes in there. So I'm not answering the question really.

Audience question read by Raymond G. Romanczyk: The next question is similar, "How do you address writing goals in domains that third party payers are less likely to fund because of categorizing the areas as educational versus medical necessity in your models?". This is a big challenge to the field in terms of educational necessity versus medical necessity.

Ronald Leaf: Yes, this is real easy one for me because I'm going to give it to Andy who does it because I don't even know what you're talking about. Andy, can you answer that one? Andy is our Psych Director and is also an attorney.

So when we are writing goals for insurance, we write goals that are consistent with the DSM diagnosis and when we are writing goals for school, we write goals that are more educationally relevant and we just make that distinction. So look closely at the DSM and look at that diagnostic criteria and that's really the best way you'll be able to make that distinction. Is that clear? Does that make sense? Rely heavily on the DSM.

Sally Rogers: You know, you can do more than that, though. For instance, DSM doesn't talk about the motor deficits in autism, I don't think. Yes, minimally. I was on the committee I should know this, but I don't. But if you have a medical report from a child and anybody talks about hypertonia, then you can bring that language into it as well, so you can use any of the language from reports from the tertiary care places that did the diagnosis or the school teams who have seen the child to also bring in the speech and language, you can put speech and language under the medical part if you're talking about dyspraxia or difficulties of those kinds of things, so you can use other medical terms, in addition to the DSM diagnosis, to bring in the health coverage aspect of it for insurance.

Audience question read by Raymond G. Romanczyk: Again this is to all presenters, "How does your model deal with the needs of children and adolescents with less intensive needs, but whose social impairments are preventing them from being successful in their community?".

Ronald Leaf: We do social groups across all ages and so we have social groups with children or adolescents and don't need intensive therapy, but can benefit from social groups. We also provide therapy for those folks, too. So we have three therapists that do therapy on an ongoing basis for adolescents who are encountering social issues in school, some adults too, so it's the social groups and therapy.

Sally Rogers: All the work I do is within 5 s, so I don't think this really applies to me. We certainly do peer work, somebody asked that, I saw, so that in our curriculum by the time kids are in level two they are in peer interactions, so we do play partners, play dates, preschool… those kinds of things. We deal with the social interactions with peers in both their home base and their preschool base, but other than that…

Mark L. Sundberg: I refer people to Crafting Connections by Mitch Taubman, Ron Leaf, and John McEachin. I think they have done some of the most excellent work in the area of social behaviors. It's awesome stuff.

William Ahearn: Yes, I would second or third that notion. I suppose the question was specifically about our models, so our model has. Wait, I'm not answering the question, I'm being just difficult. But within the context of the services that we have in public school classrooms, we are naturally serving those with lesser intensity and our extended scope and sequence goes from the most rudimentary social skills to having friends, holding jobs, and I certainly don't hope it's actually made it into Ace curriculum about asking for a date but…

John McEachin: I think you guys are all doing yourself a bit of a disservice. I think there is a very easy way to answer that question and I think it's exactly the way that we would approach treating a 3-year-old, with high- or low-level skills. The process is the same process, one of assessment, strengths and weaknesses, areas of need, and using systematic behavioral approach to teaching the skills. I think that works across all of the models, equally.

Ronald Leaf: Just to make a comment, I talked in my speech about how important social was and I think we have a love for social and a need for it, by working in the adult world. For 15 years, working with adults during institutionalization and they are coming out state hospitals with no connection, no friendships whatsoever and, through diligent work, incredible staff, friendships started occurring, meaningful relationships started occurring. We had to look at sexuality policies. These were people that couldn't care less about each other, and then 10 years later, we have to come up with sex policies because they care about each other. There are friendships occurring everywhere. When we went back to working with children, we recognized just how essential that was. When they walk in the door at 12 months of age and we get them, we've got to do the social kind of work. We have got to get the meaningful friendships and regardless of IQ, regardless of communication skills, whatever, they can have meaningful friendships and meaningful… and I think that is something that has to be defined and Mitch did a great job in the book talking about what meaningful friendships were. That's reciprocal relationships. That's not a paid friend. It's not necessarily a family friend. It's a true friendship with equal caring, reciprocity. It's absolutely essential because it's a quality-of-life issue when all is said and done because if you look at the research on isolation and depressions and suicidal ideation and suicide it is striking, alarming, and scary. So it comes down to why I had social 'screaming' in red and capitalized because it's absolutely an important element in what we need to do and it is a task analysis. I think that is the beauty of ABA, look at problem and you just have to look at the problem and figure it out and use the skills, all the wonderful skills that Mark had, those 25 or 100 skills, you have to use those skills and teach whether its sexuality or socialization or whatever it is, but socialization—you have got to focus on that.

Raymond G. Romanczyk: That brings us to an interesting point, which is 4:00 pm. To keep us on schedule, it is amazing that it is just exactly 4:00 pm, it is time to wrap up. But I have to embarrass these folk a little bit first. As we said in the beginning, this has been almost 2 years in the planning. These are extraordinary folks.

There are many individuals out there who promote different models. You know, speak a lot at conventions, who would not agree to these ground rules. To simply to come up and be colleagues in the full sense of that word, share information, look at commonalities, look at differences, look at their research, and discuss as a group. So this is really extraordinary and I have had the great pleasure of spending time with all of them as a group. And by the way, when you get them together over dinner they are hysterical. They really get along and are outstanding colleagues. So I hope you appreciate as much as I do just what they have given us today.

Ronald Leaf: And if I could just comment, if it wasn't for Ray, this wouldn't have happened. Ray deserves the applause.

Raymond G. Romanczyk: Safe travels everyone. We would love your feedback, if you would like us to do something like this again. Just go to the registration site. There is an email link. Email me and let me know that this was useful.

Chapter 9
Epilogue: ASD Treatment Implementation—Parameters and Considerations

Rachel N.S. Cavalari and Jennifer M. Gillis

One of the major challenges faced by families of individuals with ASD, especially young children, is that there are a wide variety of treatments available from both professional and non-professional providers. Although the mantra of "earlier is better" is being echoed more frequently with regard to ASD treatment, the question of what type of treatment and how much has not yet reached the same level of repetition or volume in such recitations. And yet, access to appropriate evidence-based services can have a significant impact that changes the trajectory of a child's development from that point onward. Such a cost to an individual's well-being should be of paramount concern.

Deciding what treatment to pursue can be heavily influenced by front-line professionals, such as pediatricians, nurses, or daycare providers, who might be the first professional encountered by a parent. Further, state agencies or school districts operating under Child Find mandates contained within IDEA (20 U.S.C. 1412(a)(3)) also are a source of guidance for families once a child has been identified as in need of services. However, the media and the lay public also strongly contribute to the information flow a family receives. Given this, it is necessary to disseminate accurate information about effective, evidence-based treatments to clarify the facts and dispel existing myths about these approaches. Further, in congruence with standards for evidence-based practice defined explicitly by the medical and psychological field, providers working with individuals with ASD should be actively integrating the highest standard of research evidence with clinical expertise and patient values to optimize clinical outcomes (Sackett, Rosenberg, Gray, Haynes, & Richardson, 1996). Such a standard of evidence needs to be demonstrated through

R.N.S. Cavalari, Ph.D., BCBA-D (✉)
Institute for Child Development, Binghamton University, Binghamton, NY, USA
e-mail: cavalari@binghamton.edu

J.M. Gillis, Ph.D., BCBA-D
Binghamton University, Binghamton, NY, USA
e-mail: jmattson@binghamton.edu

R.G. Romanczyk, J. McEachin (eds.), *Comprehensive Models of Autism Spectrum Disorder Treatment*, DOI 10.1007/978-3-319-40904-7_9

controlled research, including randomized clinical trials, controlled group research, and well-conducted replicated single-case methodology designs.

All of the presented models from the conference proceedings highlighted the use of controlled evaluations of their models using experimental designs noted above as forms of evidence demonstration. Given the focus population of ASD, it is not surprising that each model shares a number of similar features, including the foundations of their approaches in behavioral theory. Readers are referred to Table 9.1 for a detailed comparison of model characteristics, as shared by presenters. To summarize the similarities that extend beyond a basis in behavioral theory, all models were described as flexible, non-protocol-driven, or varied depending on the needs of the learner. This is the hallmark of individualized treatment. One year was indicated as a reliable estimate of minimum treatment duration across models given the pervasive nature of ASD. All presenters indicated that parents are integral to treatment within their model. Further, all the presented models focus on social, communication, adaptive, motor, and learning skill development, with a goal of reducing interfering or competing behavior to encourage independence. In terms of staff structure, all models reported using a hierarchical team model, with an advanced supervisor coordinating and overseeing other professional and paraprofessional team members after a minimum of 80 h of training. Despite the above similarities, targeted age ranges vary significantly between models, with the Lovaas Model and NECC focusing on early childhood through adulthood and ESDM and Verbal Behavior emphasizing early development learning skills. Service delivery setting also differed, along with a range of costs per year and intensity of service (hours per week). Data collection methods also differ, as do the methods for summarizing data to assess progress and determine when changes to treatment are needed—yet all use a data-based feedback loop, a key component of effective treatment.

As noted by the presenters, there are multiple interventions that have support in the research literature for implementation with individuals with ASD, all of which are based on the principles of applied behavior analysis, some more so than others. And yet, many presenters alluded to the challenges faced when attempting to disseminate these effective approaches due to misinformation that pervades societal understanding of what ABA truly is and what an effective program looks like. Due to these misperceptions, proponents of evidence-based methods have much work to do beyond their evidence demonstrated through research; there is also a great deal of public education and "brand" reputation management needed. If treatments were accepted into popular use based on research evidence alone, ABA-based methods would have been the norm for individuals with ASD many decades ago, without opposition.

Beyond the public perception of ABA, the pragmatics of implementation remain a very significant issue. All of the models shared in the conference proceedings estimate preliminary training of close to 100 h, with substantially more hours required to become a supervisor within an approach. Each entry-level interventionist and supervisor also require 'masters-level' supervision during their ongoing service delivery. All of these amount to substantial up-front costs and sustained supervision

Table 9.1 Comparison of evidence-based models

	Lovaas/AP[a]	ESDM[b]	NECC[c]	ABA/VB[d]
Style	Flexible, non-protocol	Flexible, non-protocol	Varied	Flexible, non-protocol
Age range	6 months through Adult[e]	9–48 months	Birth through adult	Unspecified (childhood)
Length	2+ years	1–2 years	Unspecified; varies	Unspecified; varies
Intensity (hours per week)	30	Range of 1–25	Unspecified; varies	Unspecified; varies
Setting	Clinic	Any setting natural to the child	Home and clinic	Any setting natural to the child
Cost (year)	$120,000	$50,000 (25 h/week)	$75,000–$100,000	Contract-based
Parent role	Generalization	Interventionist	Generalization	Generalization
Skill areas	• Communication	• Communication	• Discrimination skills	• Language
	• Recreation	• Relationships	• Verbal behavior	• Play
	• Coping	• Play	• Social	• Social
	• Daily living	• Joint attention	• Self-help skills	
	• Social	• Imitation	• Health and safety	
		• Motor	• Physical education	
		• Daily living	• Independence	
Staff structure	• Advanced clinical	• Team leader (any ESDM-trained professional) and parent	• Program leadership	• Supervisors
	• Mentors	• Other professional consultants	• Program specialists	• Direct care
	• Coordinators and Supervisors	• Paraprofessionals	• Frontline supervisors	
	• Direct care		• Direct care	
Initial training (hours per year)	800	80+[f]	100+	Unspecified—ABA & VB training over several years

(continued)

Table 9.1 (continued)

	Lovaas/AP[a]	ESDM[b]	NECC[c]	ABA/VB[d]
Focus and approach	• Use ABA to:	• Developmental sequences for teaching	• Use ABA to:	• Use ABA to:
	• Reduce interfering behavior	• ABA naturalistic teaching practices	• Reduce behavioral excesses	• Reduce interfering behavior
	• Teach how to learn	• FBA and behavior plan, as needed	• Develop skills to address behavioral deficits	• Develop skills
	• Develop skills	• Use of decision tree to individualize plan to child needs		
Data collection	Varied (e.g., frequency, rate, interval, time-sample)	Interval & Likert-scale	Varied (e.g., frequency, rate, interval, time-sample)	Trial-based (first trial correct mastery criteria across specified # of days)

[a]Lovaas/autism partnership
[b]Early start Denver model
[c]New England Center for Children
[d]Applied behavior analysis/verbal behavior
[e]Young autism project = not yet 4 years old at time of entry to study
[f]Didactic with 1:1 supervision over extended period of time for certification

costs over time. Added into the other costs of care, presenters estimated annual costs for their interventions between $50,000 to over $100,000. Consider the cost of service provision if these reflect only services delivered for one child. Further, although some providers are able to operate within a clinic-based structure, implementation of these models in other settings (i.e., school or home environments) or by individual practitioners presents another layer of difficulty with regard to the integrity of the model.

Even if all of the above challenges were addressed, regulations and approved parameters for service delivery vary significantly between states, provinces, and countries, as well as funding sources. In the United States, there have been ongoing discussions about who is responsible for what aspects of treatment for individuals with ASD. Specifically, decisions regarding access to care are often divided between "educational" and "medical", with approval for funding contingent on proving a demonstrated need for services to either a school district or insurance provider (Romanczyk, Callahan, Turner, & Cavalari, 2014). These somewhat arbitrary distinctions hamper access to care for individuals with ASD, limiting their ability to obtain the recommended type and intensity of treatment demonstrated as critical to progress in the evidence-based literature.

The EIBI framework, which is aimed at providing intervention for children under the age of 5 years old, has shown high levels of effectiveness for improving the developmental course for many children with ASD. The specific curricula used in evidence-based EIBI vary as is exemplified in this book. Commonalities of the interventions described in this book that have also been shown to have empirical support in treatment outcome studies benefit from trained and supervised staff, as well as parental involvement. This, sometimes, is not feasible in some service settings for a variety of reasons. First, and least likely to make an impact, is that the level of staff training or certification required might be cost-prohibitive for certain agencies or families. For example, in some states, funding of staff training opportunities might only allow for a few key staff and might not include covering the costs of continuing education credits. Some methods might not be sustainable nor pragmatic for different geographic settings (e.g., rural) or settings with fewer resources (e.g., parental pay is not feasible, lack of insurance funding, limited trained or certified therapists, etc.).

With increasing funding available to families for ASD treatment, there will be increased demand in the provision of insurance-funded interventions. Currently, 44 states have passed insurance coverage for ABA intervention for children with ASD. The demand for such services is currently outpacing the availability of such services, especially in rural areas. This gap will likely continue to widen and might ultimately lead to other interventions, with a poorer research base, to attempt to address the need for services. As researchers and practitioners who focus on the provision of evidence-based treatment for ASD, there is much at stake, especially for children with ASD and their families. It is imperative that discussions begin to identify and develop solutions that pertain to the majority of settings. The intervention approaches described in this book are excellent, yet require a level of oversight and specific set of parameters to implement properly that are simply unavailable in many settings due to state regulations concerning credentialing along with prohibitions on specifying methodology when service eligibility is determined, lack of resources, including trained or certified staff, etc. There is much at stake, and thus it is a priority to address this issue of lack of equitable access to evidence-based effective services.

As part of this effort, we need to provide parents and caregivers with guidance and information on evidence-based treatments for ASD. Not only do we as researchers in the field of ASD intervention need to do this, but also the pediatricians, nurses, early intervention staff, psychologists, and others who have primary contact with parents when a concern about their child's development or an ASD diagnosis occurs. We know that for most parents making a decision about treatment(s) for their child with ASD can be difficult for a variety of reasons. A recent article by Call, Delfs, Reavis, and Mevers (2015) highlights part of the complexity in the decision-making process for parents. On the one hand, parents showed a tendency to prefer treatments with empirical support over those with immediate effects and limited or lack of empirical support. Interestingly, if parents are selecting several treatments at once and if they have an option of significant resources, often they do not choose more of the evidence-based treatment—rather, they select even more and different treatments to implement for their child (Call et al., 2015). This should concern our field as by selecting additional interventions (with a wide range of empirical support), the dosage of effective behavioral interventions will be lessened, and as a result, the efficacy for the child reduced. Although it is unclear why this pattern of decision-making was demonstrated, it nevertheless indicates that there are multiple variables at play when selecting a treatment for a child with ASD and our field has much to do to assist parents when making these important, and sometimes life-changing, decisions. What clinicians and parents do not have available is a good decision-making algorithm, not necessarily for choosing an intervention, but more so for determining if an intervention is "working" for their child.

Recently, there is an important call of "what works for whom" (e.g., Fava & Strauss, 2014) and it is suggested that a cross-disciplinary and collaborative approach be implemented to carefully and objectively address this important question. Sometimes this notion of addressing the heterogeneity of ASD through the selection of a variety of treatments might be considered without a context, such as national autism organizations not endorsing any treatments, even those with empirical support, (Stephenson, Carter, & Kemp, 2012) which might impact a parent's decision. They may choose to select an intervention based on supposed idiosyncratic child factors rather than the principles of applied behavior analysis. While understanding factors that predict response to treatment is imperative, unfortunately, there is insufficient research currently available to help answer the question "what works for whom?" to guide parents and others in making decisions. In addition, understanding of the factors, both child characteristics and intervention methodology and parameters that might mediate treatment outcome (e.g., examination of non-responders), is needed. Perhaps a critical variable is the sequence of implementation of specific goals and how they serve to assemble repertoires of competency that allow for synergistic growth and independence.

Within the ABA behavioral framework, one can begin to address "what works for whom" as each intervention addressing specific child needs is highly individualized such that no child receives a cookie-cutter program. Thus, no one child should receive the same set of teaching targets or behavioral targets. The process of ongoing assessment, data collection, and analysis allows practitioners to identify when a procedure is or is NOT working, further allowing for refinement of a child's intervention program or approach. At a minimum, practitioners who are Board-Certified Behavior Analysts are apt to apply a more rigorous examination of *any* intervention with the application of single case designs, and it is this strength that would allow for a more objective exploration of "what works for whom."

Research needs to continue to address this question of what works in the sense of how evidence-based treatments are individualized for a given child. But funding needs to be available now to allow for the examination of innovative models for implementation of evidence-based interventions, such as those covered in this book, that do not sacrifice or compromise efficacy. Examining ways to more efficiently train therapists, educators, parents, and staff to implement these interventions is vitally important as one component of bringing services to scale and reducing costs.

There is great work to be done as we all forge ahead. It is critical that researchers involved in treatment outcome research in ASD work together to allow for a better dissemination of these treatments to consumers and other professionals. Further, emphasis must be placed on investigating potentially critical individual and treatment variables in order to meet the goals of increased access to evidence-based treatments for more individuals with ASD across the lifespan.

References

Call, N. A., Delfs, C. H., Reavis, A. R., & Mevers, J. L. (2015). Factors influencing treatment decisions by parents for their children with autism spectrum disorder. *Research in Autism Spectrum Disorders, 15*, 10–20.

Fava, L., & Strauss, K. (2014). Response to early intensive behavioral intervention for autism—An umbrella approach to issues critical to treatment individualization. *International Journal of Developmental Neuroscience, 39*, 49–58.

Romanczyk, R. G., Callahan, E. H., Turner, L. B., & Cavalari, R. N. S. (2014). Efficacy of behavioral interventions for young children with autism spectrum disorders: Public policy, the evidence base, and implementation parameters. *Review Journal of Autism and Developmental Disorders, 1*(4), 276–326. doi:10.1007/s40489-014-0025-6.

Sackett, D. L., Rosenberg, W. M., Gray, J. A., Haynes, R. B., & Richardson, W. S. (1996). Evidence based medicine: What it is and what it isn't. *British Medical Journal, 312*(7023), 71–72.

Stephenson, J., Carter, M., & Kemp, C. (2012). Quality of the information on educational and therapy interventions provided on the web sites of national autism associations. *Research in Autism Spectrum Disorders, 6*(1), 11–18.

Index

R.G. Romanczyk, J. McEachin (eds.), *Comprehensive Models of Autism Spectrum Disorder Treatment*, DOI 10.1007/978-3-319-40904-7

MIX
Papier aus verantwortungsvollen Quellen
Paper from responsible sources
FSC® C105338

If you have any concerns about our products,
you can contact us on
ProductSafety@springernature.com

In case Publisher is established outside the EU,
the EU authorized representative is:
Springer Nature Customer Service Center GmbH
Europaplatz 3, 69115 Heidelberg, Germany

Printed by Libri Plureos GmbH
in Hamburg, Germany